The ABC's of Prenatal Diagnosis

A Guide to Pregnancy Testing and Issues

BY KEITH & LAURIE WEXLER

EDITED BY PAUL WEXLER, M.D., F.A.C.O.G.

Clinical Professor Department of OB/GYN at
The University of Colorado Health Sciences Center

GENASSIST PUBLISHING INC.
Denver, CO

Dedicated to our beautiful daughter,
Haylee Erin Wexler

To our parents, Nick and Linda, and Paul and Hilde
for encouraging us to ask questions.

Special Thanks To:
Kathie, Sherry, Dr. Abrams, Michael, Troy, Emma, Alice, Jeremy,
Laura, Jen, Jane, Anne, Mark, Kent and Debbie, Patrick, Jamie,
Chance, Amanda, T.J. and Laura, Susan and John,
Adam, Charlie.

Designed by David Schmidt, Studio 2 Graphic Arts, Ltd.
Denver, CO

FOREWORD

During our first pregnancy my wife, Laurie, established a policy that I was permitted to worry about only one thing per day. However, no restriction was placed on how much I could worry about each issue.

This might seem a trivial point but we have noticed that most of our friends who are pregnant now and those who have been recently pregnant worry about the health and welfare of their future child.

There was not a single day from the pre-planning of the pregnancy to the first breath that our child, Haylee Erin, took in the delivery room that Laurie and I were not reading books and asking questions to make sure we gave our baby the best chance for a happy and healthy future. This quest for answers to our myriad of questions led to this book.

It is a compilation of those questions and answers that Laurie and I posed to our health care professionals. To be able to access the information, we have listed the subjects covered in alphabetical order. These subjects are options that are available to you whether or not your health care professional offers them to you or not. Although it might not be necessary for every pregnant mother to have access to all of the latest technology, we, like most expectant parents, wanted to be aware of the technology so that we could choose the direction that would give our child the best chance at a healthy future.

The questions and answers should not be taken to represent all the questions that could or should be asked. The answers do not represent all the possible answers, only those given to us by our health care professionals. It merely is a list of questions and answers that made up our evolution to first time parenting. We have sought and continue to encourage input from other parents or expectant parents and think of this as an ongoing project in search of questions and answers.

We hope this layout of our thought process will help encourage and inspire other parents to ask what is on their mind. We are not born knowing how to be parents and we must educate ourselves and hope that the answers we find are the right ones.

I end with a quote that my father, Paul Wexler, M.D. (an OB/GYN doctor) and my mother, Hilde Wexler, (a former hospital administrator) impressed upon my wife and me:

"Never be afraid to ask your health care professional questions that concern you. We in the health care field can only answer the questions you ask, not the questions you are thinking about."

Keith Wexler

PREFACE

At no other time in our lives does the responsibility for getting answers to our questions weigh so heavily as when we undertake a decision to bear or adopt a child. The responsibility to give your child the best start and the greatest opportunities carries over from early childhood into adulthood.

As an obstetrician-gynecologist for more than 25 years, my enthusiasm for answering many of the same questions over and over again never dampened since each patient or couple demonstrated the same enthusiasm for the answers. This search for answers led Laurie and Keith to read as much as they could digest and then ask for input from their parents, friends and health care providers.

Keith and Laurie were surprised to learn of the great diversity of care and sharing of information which occurred with different health care givers. They felt committed to getting the information out about the new technology available to couples today. Not all of these advances have been positive as often the technology may raise more questions than it answers. Yet, despite these limitations, Keith and Laurie felt that as consumers of health care and prospective parents they were entitled to have the information. Often, the health care giver feels the need to filter the information given to a patient to achieve a preconceived goal. With the explosion of information, particularly medical information, a plan to restrict access to information even if for a "loftier" goal will invariably lead to continued distrust of the health care provider. As health care providers, we should accept the challenge to get answers for our patients and ourselves.

The medical editing of the information has been done with great care to avoid diluting the information with unnecessary medical detail yet attempting to assure the accuracy. The foreword sets forth that there are no correct answers to the questions asked, only opinions. These opinions can be used to gather information from your health care giver. Thus, the responsibility for deciding to start or raise a family can be shared with the professionals committed to similar goals. Such shared responsibility should lighten the "burden of childbearing" and change it into the exciting miracle of birth and child rearing that a Haylee Erin in your life should be.

Paul Wexler, M.D.

Table of Contents

Foreword
Preface

AMNIOCENTESIS (Amnio)

AMNIOTIC BANDS

BETA HCG - SERUM HUMAN CHORIONIC GONADOTROPIN (HCG)

BLOOD CHROMOSOMES

CHROMOSOMAL ABNORMALITIES

(CVS) CHORIONIC VILLUS SAMPLING

The ABC's Of Prenatal Diagnosis Order Form

ABC's of Pregnancy

a. Once you are pregnant, then what?

When we made the decision to have a baby, we never realized how many decisions we would need to make during the pregnancy. We thought the hardest part would be picking out a name and finishing the nursery. The decision to get pregnant was the easiest, although getting pregnant is not always easy. Once I found out that I was in fact pregnant, I became concerned with my eating and drinking habits. I did not want to be responsible for adversely affecting the health and well-being of the child growing inside of me. Many pregnant mothers that we have talked with want the pregnancy to simply be a joyous experience and can not bear to deal with the reality that there might be a problem with a pregnancy. Denial is normal for such a beautiful thing as pregnancy. However, decisions that you make or do not make during the pregnancy will have an impact on the child for at least 21 years while he/she is under your care. People talk all the time of investing in their child's future but we too often give lip service rather than doing what we know is right.

Since each pregnancy and each baby is unique, an expectant mother or couple must make decisions that are right for them and the pregnancy. Each expectant mother or couple will be faced with a new set of decisions for each pregnancy. After speaking with several of our friends that live in other states, we quickly came to realize that prenatal care varies amongst health care providers. Each state has its own accepted standard of care, and each health care provider has tests that he/she likes or dislikes. Medical providers are human and do have biases in favor of or against certain techniques and technology. This does not make it right or wrong, but it is something to be aware of during your prenatal care. The testing that was offered to us was not universally offered to all of our friends, and our friends were offered testing that we were never offered.

The tests that we had performed during the pregnancy were in hopes of doing all we could to give our child the healthiest entry into the world. We considered every advantage and disadvantage that the testing and the test results would have on our pregnancy. We were given free access to the information and were allowed to make an educated decision based upon facts. We feel that every expectant mother or couple should have access to this information, and be able to make decisions affecting their pregnancy in the privacy of their own home. Helping other expectant mothers or couples become educated consumers is what led to this book. No matter whether you are pregnant or not, old or young, adopted or an infertility patient, it is never too early to prepare for a pregnancy.

This book hopefully will act as an alphabetical guide to obtaining the information that you will need during the pregnancy. The tests and concepts discussed in this book are by no means a national standard of care, nor should you run to your health care provider and force him/her to practice medicine differently because of this book. It is a guide to help take some of the mystery out of medicine and prenatal diagnosis. Each expectant mother's or couples' family history, personal medical history, and attitudes are going to influence what will be the right course of action for their baby. The decisions that we made during our pregnancy may have been very different from what our friends did or would have done, but it was right for us and our baby. We hope everyone has the same access to information and opportunities to make those decisions.

ADOPTION

(Most of what we know in the field of Genetics, we learn from looking at the patient and/or couple)

a. How do I assess my genetic risks if I am adopted?

Most patients who were adopted pose a medical history problem for the field of genetics. Since most adoptees have little to no information regarding their biological parents, any genetic predisposition that might be found in that family is usually lost. The adoptee who has an interest in getting family information should contact the adoption agency or have a parent contact the agency to get any information which is available. However, most adoptees will have very limited success in getting much information. There is currently no national movement to make this information available.

When your history is not available, the best way to evaluate your fetus' possible risk is to review your own personal medical history and that of your partner. In the absence of historical family information, your family history can begin with you. If only one of the couple is adopted, you can begin your family tree with the family history of the non-adopted individual. Remember, adoption alone does not place you at a greater risk for problems with your own children. Although having an accurate family history can assist in anticipating risks for recurrence in other family members, the lack of such historical information does not preclude risk assessment of any pregnancy. It has been our observation that most people who choose prenatal diagnosis get little or no family history from other family members even if they are still alive. The reason seems to be that most individuals do not like to talk about relatives with problems.

Each newborn baby is a new generation of genetic information; each relative that dies takes a generation of history with him or her. Often, family members can be encouraged to share information, even negative information, if they believe the interest in this information grows out of true concern. The adoptee can keep a detailed history of his/her own and his/her partner's medical history so that as their children grow they can learn about their parents' history. The general population risk for having a child with a birth defect is approximately 3%-5%. A positive family history increases this risk. The risks assessment of an adoptee can be based on:

1. Chronological age of mother and father.
2. How many children mother and father have had?
3. Were all of the pregnancies normal? If not, what problems did they have?
4. Ethnic/Racial background of mother and father.
5. Miscarriages/Ectopic pregnancies.
6. Drugs taken at the time of conception or during pregnancy.
7. The status of the current pregnancy. Were there illnesses in early pregnancy?
8. Medical history since childhood for the adoptee.

b. Is there a "general screen" that is available for adoptees?

Doctors would love to have a single test for all individuals in which a blood specimen could be tested to tell whether the adoptee is a carrier, affected or free of a particular disease or trait. However, no such test exists and the prospect for such a screen is not in the foreseeable future.

Adoptee Testing: Currently an individual or a couple planning a pregnancy or who are currently pregnant have some Prenatal Diagnostic choices:

1. Maternal serum AFP/AFP2/AFP3 (See AFP Chapter).
2. An ultrasound survey of the fetus, amniotic fluid, uterus and placenta.
3. Chromosome Analysis - Blood chromosomes on parents before pregnancy to help rule out a chromosomal abnormality in one or both parents. In the absence of a prior abnormal pregnancy or two or more miscarriages, the probability of an abnormal finding is small.
4. Selective DNA testing on mother and/or father based upon Ethnic/Racial background: i.e Cystic Fibrosis (Caucasian), Tay Sachs (Jewish Ethnicity), Thalassemia (Italian/Asian) or Sickle Cell Anemia (Black Ancestry).
5. CVS/Early Amniocentesis/Amniocentesis - To help rule out a chromosomal abnormality in the fetus.

(AFP) ALPHAFETOPROTEIN

a. What is AFP?

AFP is the abbreviation for alphafetoprotein. Alphafetoprotein is a protein released by the fetus into the amniotic fluid while it is developing during the pregnancy. The level of AFP can be used to help monitor the well being of the fetus. Between 14 and 22 weeks gestation, the AFP level of the fetus can be analyzed simply by removing blood from the mother, since the fetus' AFP travels through the mother's blood stream. AFP levels that are elevated can help identify or help rule out most open neural tube or gastrointestinal wall defects in the fetus. AFP levels that are decreased can help identify possible chromosomal problems in the fetus, particularly Down syndrome.

b. What causes AFP to be high or low?

Some conditions which cause high or elevated AFP levels in the blood of the pregnant mother include:

1. Multiple gestations (twins, triplets, etc.)
2. Large infants.
3. Due dates that are earlier than expected.
4. Known or unknown bleeding inside the uterus.
5. Rarely, problems with the pregnancy or fetus such as kidney or intestinal problems, problems with brain or spinal cord development, openings in the abdomen muscle which covers the intestines or chromosomal problems.

It is important to remember that maternal blood AFP is a **screening** test only. An abnormal test result does not mean that your baby is not normal. Most patients with high or elevated AFP levels have a perfectly normal baby. Since an elevated AFP may indicate a problem with your pregnancy or baby, your health care professional will probably want you to have a thorough ultrasound study to confirm gestational dates and look at the development of the fetus.

Your health care provider might suggest repeating the AFP test to double check the values. If the value is still elevated, you may be asked to meet with a genetic specialist to discuss options of further testing (e.g. amniocentesis in which a needle is placed in the bag of water surrounding the fetus in order to obtain amniotic fluid for more specific testing).

Some conditions that can cause blood AFP to be low include:

1. A due date later than expected.
2. Rarely, problems with the pregnancy such as a miscarriage, which has not yet passed, or Down syndrome.

It is important to remember that blood AFP is a **screening** test only. An abnormal test result does not mean that your baby is not normal. Most patients with low AFP have a perfectly normal baby. Since low AFP may indicate a problem with the pregnancy or fetus, your health care provider will probably suggest that you have a thorough ultrasound study to confirm dates and look at the physiology of the fetus. Your health care professional might suggest that you have another AFP run to confirm the value. If the value is still low you might be referred to a genetic specialist to discuss options of further testing.

1. How high is high, how low is low?

AFP values are reported as high, low or normal. Most laboratories consider a normal range of 0.50 Multiples of the Median (MoM's) to 2.0 MoM's on maternal blood. If the AFP comes back at 2.01 MoM's or greater it must be read as a high or elevated result. If the value comes back 0.49 MoM's or lower it must be read as low.

c. Why is the AFP abnormal this pregnancy if it was normal last pregnancy?

Just because this pregnancy's AFP level is abnormal when it was normal before (in previous pregnancies) is not anything to become alarmed about. Each pregnancy and each fetus develops uniquely and the AFP levels of the fetus will vary from pregnancy to pregnancy. Since most women who are under the age of 35 years of age are not routinely offered prenatal diagnostic testing, AFP is a relatively inexpensive ($30-$50) and non-invasive way to evaluate the fetus. It is hard for the expectant mother and partner to ignore an abnormal AFP value, whether high or low. There is current testing available to determine that there is nothing physically or chromosomally wrong with the fetus.

In the past two years, the AFP normal range has become narrower, moving from (0.50 MoM's - 2.5 MoM's) to (0.50 MoM's - 2.0 MoM's). The rationale for decreasing the "normal range" is that it should help catch abnormalities that were missed in the larger "normal" range. It also means that there is a greater chance of false positives (babies that test positive, but are normal). The biggest problem with AFP screening is not the false positives, since they can be ruled out by current testing; rather it is the false negatives that are missed. Just because your AFP level is abnormal does not mean that there is anything wrong with your fetus. Likewise, just because your AFP test is normal does not mean that the baby will not have any problems. This "false negative" group has caused consumers to push for tougher guidelines for laboratories to help catch affected babies not picked up by this test.

d. If the AFP is abnormal this pregnancy will it be abnormal for all subsequent pregnancies?

A high or low AFP value in one pregnancy does not mean that it will be abnormal in a subsequent pregnancy. AFP levels are fetus specific, and the development of the fetus and pregnancy dictate what AFP levels are released. A patient can have one pregnancy with a high AFP, a second pregnancy with a low AFP, and a third pregnancy with a normal AFP. We decided early in our pregnancy that, for our sanity, we would only worry about those tests that returned abnormal, rather than worry about the tests that might. Like the old proverb says, "if you wish for something hard enough it probably will come true".

e. What is AFP2 and AFP3?

AFP2 is the combination of two tests, alphafetoprotein and beta human chorionic gonadotropin or pregnancy hormone (HCG) to enhance the detection of trisomy 21 (Down syndrome) fetuses in women under the age of 35. At the time of this publication, only 20%-30% of infants with trisomy 21 (Down syndrome) are born to women who are 35 or older. Low maternal serum AFP and an elevated beta HCG used together can help identify 50%-55% of fetuses with trisomy 21 who might have otherwise escaped detection.

AFP3 - Also called the tri-screen or triple screen, is a combination of AFP, beta HCG and Estriol. Although each of the reagents have independently been approved by the FDA, the reagents used in combination with one another for AFP3 screening is still considered investigational by the FDA and most laboratories that perform the test. Recent literature claims a detection rate of 89% for trisomy 21 (Down syndrome) using AFP3 in women over age 35. Other studies report only a 60%-70% reliability for detection of Down syndrome when pregnant women of all ages were studied. Therefore at least 11% of

Down syndrome babies will not be detected. Also, approximately 50% of other chromosome abnormalities will not be detected with this test. **Patients that have a normal AFP3 have not had their fetuses tested for Down syndrome.** AFP3 is only a screening test that helps identify pregnancies that are at a greater risk for Down syndrome. Under current technology the only way to verify that a fetus has Down syndrome is to perform a CVS, early amniocentesis or amniocentesis.

Recommendations for AFP3: All women who formerly were candidates for prenatal diagnosis should still be offered prenatal diagnostic testing, whether the AFP3 test is positive or negative.

1. AFP3 can only be done on patients between 15 and 21.9 weeks gestation because at present there are no values for comparison prior to or after these weeks. AFP3 can only be performed on maternal serum - (mother's blood), not on amniotic fluid. Elevated maternal serum AFP, even as part of AFP3 must be followed up to help identify possible open neural tube and/or abdominal wall defects. A high maternal serum AFP result should be repeated to confirm results.
2. AFP3 is most valuable when combined with ultrasound to confirm gestational dates.
3. AFP3 is a screening test only. **It does not test whether or not your baby has Down syndrome.**
4. Results for an AFP3 may take as long as 7-14 days.
5. When your health care professional receives the AFP3 result, both the risk for Down syndrome and the alphafetoprotein results must be reviewed. Not simply one or the other.
6. Although AFP3 can help detect up to 89% of Down syndrome fetuses and 33%-44% of other trisomies, the test still has a false positive and/or false negative rate of 11% and 56%-66% respectively.
7. If your AFP3 is normal your baby has not been tested to see if it has Down syndrome. The only way to confirm whether a baby has Down syndrome is by performing a CVS, early amniocentesis or amniocentesis.
8. Maternal serum AFP should continue to be used as a general screening tool to help identify structural

abnormalities of the spinal canal and abdominal wall. Patients with AFP values which suggest an increased risk for chromosomal abnormalities should be offered further genetic counseling and possible additional prenatal diagnostic testing.

f. Does every pregnant mother have to have an AFP?

No pregnant mother can be forced to submit to testing that she elects not to have performed. There are a growing number of states that are requiring that all pregnant mothers must be offered some type of AFP screening between 14 and 22 weeks gestation. In some states, if a mother refuses testing she will be asked to sign a consent form that she was apprized of the risk for birth defects and has elected not to have the test performed. She may be asked to waive her right to sue the doctor, hospital, insurance company or state in the event that a baby has a physical and/or chromosomal abnormality.

In most states, a woman has the ultimate right to decide what will and will not be done to her own body during pregnancy. However, more states are adopting AFP testing as a general screening tool which is non-invasive to the fetus. Some states are drafting legislation which places more of the financial burden for supporting the child on a woman who chooses not to have testing. This ethical and moral dilemma of "patient responsiblity" is still in its infancy stage but is gaining momentum in legislative, political and medical circles as the issue of health care reform is debated.

g. What is the difference between maternal serum AFP (MS-AFP) and amniotic fluid AFP (AF-AFP)?

MS-AFP is a screening test performed on a mother's blood to see if the fetus' AFP level is high, low or normal during the pregnancy. The MS-AFP can help identify possible problems with the fetus, but does not pinpoint exactly what's wrong. It is a red flag that tells us that something **may** be wrong. An abnormal result simply means that the health care professional must study the pregnancy carefully to try to rule out or identify a problem.

AF-AFP is performed on the amniotic fluid versus mother's blood. Since the fetus releases AFP directly into the amniotic fluid as it develops, the AFP value in the amniotic fluid is more indicative of the real level produced versus the levels found in the mother's blood stream. An AF-AFP that is low does not help much as a diagnostic procedure since the problems that are associated with a low AF-AFP value can be ruled out by a chromosome analysis of the amniotic fluid. Unlike MS-AFP, if the amniotic fluid AFP comes back elevated, the amniotic fluid can be tested to help pinpoint small open neural tube or gastrointestinal wall defects or a small bleed from the fetus to the mother. **This test does not help identify closed neural tube defects.** The only way to get amniotic fluid currently is to perform an amniocentesis.

h. My amniotic fluid AFP (AF-AFP) result is elevated. What is Acetylcholinesterase (AChE) and why is the test performed?

When an amniotic fluid AFP test is reported as elevated, 2.0 Multiples of the Median (MoM's) or higher, The College of Pathologists (CAP) who establish recommendations for most laboratories in the United States recommend that acetylcholinesterase (AChE) be performed to help identify why the AFP might be elevated. AChE is an enzyme that is released by the fetus into the amniotic fluid as the fetus develops. The AChE test can help identify possible structural abnormalities of the fetus since neural tube enzymes can be differentiated from gastrointestinal enzymes. The AChE test can help distinguish whether the elevated AF-AFP is due to:

1. An open neural tube defect.
2. An intestinal wall defect.
3. A maternal bleed or contamination of the specimen.

A negative test for AChE helps rule out most of these defects.

The use of amniotic fluid AFP testing has allowed labs that might not have seen the patient to help identify structural problems in the fetus that might have gone undetected during the ultrasound or help confirm ultrasound findings. The test usually costs an additional $75-$135 over the amniocentesis price. Having identified a structural abnormality, the health care provider can prepare for the delivery of the child, by making the delivery as safe and as non-traumatic as possible, as well as allowing time for the family to meet with neonatal specialists and surgeons to prepare for corrective surgery.

AGE - MATERNAL / PATERNAL

a. What is an age related risk for pregnancy?

Since approximately 1972 when amniocentesis first became available for prenatal diagnosis for genetic testing, the basis for recommending the procedure was based upon the theory that since a woman is born with all the eggs she will have in her lifetime she will have a greater chance of having a child with a chromosome abnormality as she ages. (Table 1) illustrates the percentage of babies born with a chromosome abnormality for every 100 pregnancies in that group. The 35 year old has an asterisk (*) because this was selected by the American College of OB/GYN as the age at which patients need to be offered prenatal diagnosis by CVS, early amniocentesis or amniocentesis because the patient has a greater risk of having an abnormality than miscarrying from the procedure.

(TABLE 1)

Maternal age (year)	Approximate risk (%)
< 20	0.05-0.08
20-24	0.08-0.10
25-29	0.08-0.15
30-34	0.12-0.20
*35-39	0.30-0.80
40-42	0.90-1.50
43-45	1.50-3.00
46-49	2.00-10.00

What does the risk of a 35 year old equate to in the probability of having an affected child?

The risk for a 35 year old woman having a child with a chromosomal abnormality is approximately 1:270. This risk is called an age-related risk because the risk for a chromosome abnormality increases as the woman gets older. The reason that women 35 years or older are at a greater risk of having an abnormality is:

1. Women are born with all of the eggs that they will require during their lifetime.
2. As the mother ages the eggs age.

3. As the eggs age, unequal separation of the chromosomes during cellular division may occur. This can cause too many or too few chromosomes to move to one cell at the time of or shortly following conception.
4. All pregnant mothers who are screened during a pregnancy will be compared with the risk of a 35 year old woman. Every pregnancy will have a risk less than, equal to or greater than 1:270.
5. Women who have a risk greater than 1:270 are usually offered prenatal diagnosis including CVS, early amniocentesis and amniocentesis.

Example #1:

A 20 year old pregnant female has no family history of genetic disease and has an AFP or AFP3 test done at 15 weeks gestation. The AFP test result returns as normal. This patient would not routinely be offered genetic amniocentesis since her risk for having a child with Down syndrome is less than a 35 year old. Also, her risk for having a child with an open neural tube defect or abdominal wall defect is not increased. All pregnancies have a 3%-5% risks for having a child with a birth defect. Her age related risk is not any greater than the general population risk for a defect. Her risk for a child with a chromosome abnormality is 0.08%-0.10%.

Example #2:

A 20 year old pregnant female has no family history of genetic disease. At 15 weeks gestation she has an AFP or AFP3 test performed. When the results come back it gives her a Down syndrome risk of 1:220. Since the risk for a 35 year old is 1:270, this patient would be offered genetic amniocentesis since her Down syndrome risk is greater than that of a 35 year old.

Example #3:

A 20 year old pregnant female has a brother with Down syndrome. The rest of her history and her partner's family history is not genetically noteworthy. What is her risk for having an affected baby?
Answer: To solve this problem the health care professional would go to (Table I) and get an age related risk for a 20

year old (0.08%-0.10%). The recurrence risk for an individual with a first degree relative with Down syndrome is approximately 1%.

Add 0.08%-0.10% to 1.0% and you get a risk of approximately 1.08%-1.10%. Look at (Table 1). This risk equates to the risk for a 40-42 year old. This patient's risk is greater than a 35 year old. Therefore, she would be offered CVS, early amniocentesis or amniocentesis.

These examples help illustrate how a recommendation for further genetic testing is determined. Since health care professionals do not have a cystal ball that can tell them which pregnancies are abnormal and which are not, this statistical analysis can help identify patients that might be at an increased risk for an abnormality.

b. What is maternal age?

Maternal age simply refers to the particular age of a pregnant woman. Insurance companies and health care professionals use maternal age to help identify women at increased risk either for having an abnormal baby or pregnancy complications.

c. What is paternal age?

While most insurance companies and health care professionals recognize maternal age over 35 years as having some increased risk for child bearing, paternal age (the age of the father of the child) is not universally recognized. Some studies have shown that men over 45 years of age are at a greater risk of having a child with a chromosomal abnormality regardless of the mother's age. Other studies have not confirmed this finding. Men over age 35 years may have an increased risk for the sudden appearance of an abnormality in their newborn which has not occurred in the family before. While most insurance companies will take the age of the biological father into consideration, it is not usually considered a reason for prenatal diagnosis.

AMNIOCENTESIS

a. What is amniocentesis? What are the indications and risks associated with an amnio?

Amniocentesis consists of inserting a needle through the pregnant women's abdomen or vagina into the sac of fluid (bag of water) surrounding the fetus. It is then possible to withdraw some of the amniotic fluid in which the baby's cells are suspended. Within the fluid are live cells from the skin of the fetus, umbilical cord, placenta and inner surface of the amniotic sac, and cells from the baby's urinary and respiratory tracts. From these cells chromosomes may be identified. This makes it possible to diagnose a number of disorders before birth. Part of the chromosome analysis involves sex determination. You **should** be asked at the time of the procedure whether or not you want to know the sex of the baby. In addition to chromosome analysis, biochemical tests and DNA tests can be run on the amniotic fluid. Your family history determines which if any of the additional tests should be performed. (See DNA Chapter)

After 14 weeks gestation, (calculated from the first day of the last menstrual period), the amniotic fluid that is removed will be tested for the presence of alphafetoprotein. This protein may be elevated in up to 90% of all pregnancies in which the fetus has an open spinal defect (e.g. spina bifida). This protein may be elevated in other conditions including inaccurate dates (i.e. number of weeks pregnant), some defects in the fetus' abdominal wall muscles or pregnancies which may be at a higher risk for miscarriage. Although normal values are being established for blood and amniotic fluid alphafetoprotein studies performed prior to 14 weeks gestation, the values are currently not believed to be reliable. Therefore, testing prior to 14 weeks may not allow for open spinal defects to be detected. When reliable tests do become available these tests should be routinely performed. (See AFP Chapter)

THE AMNIOCENTESIS PROCEDURE - TRANSABDOMINAL

The procedure of amniocentesis should include the following sequence of events:

1. An informed consent explaining the risks of the procedure is discussed and signed by the patient.

2. An optimal location for the amniocentesis is chosen with ultrasound versus performing the procedure without ultrasound guidance.

3. The site is chosen and marked on the abdomen, and washed with an antibacterial solution to cleanse the skin.

4. A small amount of local anesthesia is placed in the skin, which may be slightly uncomfortable. Some physicians perform the procedure without local anesthesia. You may wish to discuss this with your health care provider. The tissue beneath the skin is also numbed with the anesthetic solution.

5. A very thin needle is then placed through the anesthetized area through the uterus into the amniotic sac. The uterus is a thick wall of muscle, and you may feel pressure and temporary cramping. You should feel no additional cramping once the needle is in place.

6. Approximately 1 1/2 tablespoons (18 cc's) or less of fluid is removed. The total procedure usually takes less than 10 minutes.

7. After the amniocentesis procedure, the ultrasound machine will be used to show you that the baby was not harmed during the procedure.

INSTRUCTIONS FOR THE DAY OF THE AMNIOCENTESIS

1. Eat normally the day of the procedure. **Do not fast.**

2. Drink 12-36 oz of liquid (not milk) (depending upon the ultrasound machine that is used) 45 minutes prior to your scheduled amniocentesis appointment.

3. Try not to empty your bladder, as it is easier to visualize the fetus and perform the amniocentesis with a full bladder. If you must relieve some pressure, urinate only until comfortable.

4. If your bladder is not full enough for your appointment you may have to be rescheduled.

5. If an adequate pocket of fluid can not be located, or you are too early by gestational weeks, or the baby is not in an optimum position, you may be asked to return in a few days to complete the amniocentesis.

6. After completion of the amniocentesis, you may resume your normal activities. Minimize physical activities (such as heavy lifting or sports)) and rest if you have cramping.

POSSIBLE INDICATIONS FOR AMNIOCENTESIS

1. You are a pregant woman over 35 years of age or are younger than age 20.
2. You are a woman with a history of having a previous child with an abnormality (e.g. spinal defect, multiple defects or a chromosomal abnormality).
3. You are a woman with a history of two or more spontaneous miscarriages.
4. You or your partner has a history of a diagnosable, inherited abnormality in either your family or that of your partner, in a grandparent, parent, brother or sister, niece or nephew, aunt or uncle or first or second cousin.
5. You or your partner is a carrier of or is affected by a sex-linked disorder (e.g. Duchenne Muscular Dystrophy, Hemophilia).
6. You or your partner are carriers of an inborn error of metabolism (e.g. Tay Sachs, PKU/Phenylketonuria).
7. You or your partner has a serious medical disease which increases your risk for having a baby with a diagnosable abnormality (e.g. Diabetes).
8. You are a man over 45 years of age and your partner is pregnant.
9. You had an abnormal prenatal test (e.g. AFP/alpha-fetoprotein, AFP2, or AFP3 or ultrasound).
10. You or your partner is a carrier of an abnormality on one of your chromosomes.

RISK FROM AMNIOCENTESIS

1. There is a 1:200 to 1:500 (0.20%-0.50%) risk of miscarriage following the amniocentesis procedure.
2. There is a slight risk of leakage of amniotic fluid which might be blood tinged following the procedure. This leakage occurs approximately 1% of the time and is not considered a serious complication. However, your health care professional should be notified.

3. You may experience a few uterine contractions the day of the procedure and should reduce your activities for the remainder of the day.
4. As with all surgical procedures, there is a slight risk of infection. Every precaution is taken to prevent this.
5. There is a possibility (usually less than 1:100) that amniotic cells will fail to grow and the procedure will have to be repeated.

b. When can you do amniocentesis?

An amniocentesis whether done transabdominally (via the abdomen) or transvaginally (via the vagina) can be performed as early as 11 to 12 weeks gestation. The reason that amniocentesis can not performed earlier is because there is not enough amniotic fluid produced to sample safely before 11 weeks gestation. There are two factors that must be met in order to perform a "safe" amniocentesis procedure.

1. There must be enough amniotic fluid to safely remove 6-10 cc's before 14 weeks gestation and 10-16 cc's 14.1 weeks or later. If there is too little fluid (oligohydramnios) then the health care professional performing the procedure will wait until there is enough "extra" fluid to sample safely. The amniotic fluid that is removed is usually replaced by the body within 12-24 hours following the procedure.
2. The health care professional should have adequate technology (ultrasound) to visualize the fetus during the amniocentesis to locate a safe entry point to remove the fluid and to visualize the fetus to help avoid trauma to the fetus.

Early amniocentesis is performed between 11 and 14 weeks gestation. Traditional amniocentesis can be performed between 14.1 weeks and 23.5 weeks gestation in the doctor's office. After 25 weeks gestation, the procedure is usually performed in the hospital since a 25-26 week fetus may be capable of supporting its own life outside of the mother. Most states have medical technology that can save many fetuses that might deliver following the procedure .

Early amniocentesis is only performed between 11 and 14 weeks gestation because most pregnancies will have enough amniotic fluid in this time frame to perform a chromosomal analysis (to look at the number of chromosomes of the fetus and the physical integrity of the chromosomes). The difference between early amniocentesis and traditional amniocentesis is that after 14.1 weeks gestation, confirmed by ultrasound, a chromosome analysis and an amniotic fluid AFP test can be done. Before 14.1 weeks the AFP test can not be done since there are no nationally accepted values. The AFP test can help identify open neural tube or gastrointestinal wall defects that might not have been seen on ultrasound.

After 23 weeks gestation an amniotic fluid AFP is usually not performed on the fluid since there are no nationally accepted values. Many amniocentesis programs across the country choose 16 to 17 weeks gestation as the most optimal time to perform the procedure since an amniotic fluid AFP, a chromosome analysis and a Level II ultrasound (a targeted biophysical profile study of the fetus) can all be performed at the same time. Prior to 16 weeks gestation the fetus is too small to adequately study the physical integrity of the fetus.

c. Who performs the amniocentesis - a doctor or a paraprofessional?

Currently amniocentesis is only performed by a medical doctor (M.D.) or a doctor of osteopathy (D.O.) since the procedure is invasive and is considered a surgical procedure. Although, most of the people who are involved in the amniocentesis procedure are paraprofessionals (i.e. the counsellor, the nurse, the lab technicians, the ultrasound technicians etc.) all of their work must be overseen and interpreted by an M.D. or D.O. Like any surgical procedure you should ask how many procedures that doctor has performed. You should also ask what the miscarriage risk is for that doctor.

Since many pregnant women see an obstetrician/gynecologist (OB/GYN) during the pregnancy, most OB/GYN's have traditionally performed the amniocentesis. But amniocentesis can be performed by any M.D. or D.O. who has special training and feels competent to perform the procedure. Most M.D.'s have chosen not to get the special training and have usually deferred the procedure to genetic and amniocentesis specialists in their part of the country. This is not mandated by law. It is simply a conscious decision made by most doctors.

d. Is there a Board Certification for a doctor to perform CVS, early amniocentesis or amniocentesis?

Contrary to popular belief among the general population there is **NO** medical board that specifically licenses a doctor to perform CVS, early amniocentesis or amniocentesis. Amniocentesis is a surgical procedure like any other surgery (i.e. hysterectomy, tubal ligation etc.). This requires that an M.D. or D.O. have enough special training to "competently" perform the procedure. Most of the doctors who perform CVS, early amniocentesis and amniocentesis are Board Certified OB/GYN's. Another large group of amniocentesis providers are Board Certified Perinatologists.

e. Who produces amniotic fluid - me or my baby?

The answer is both. The amniotic fluid is produced in part by the amniotic fluid membranes as well as by the fetal kidney and respiratory tract. The reason a doctor monitors the amniotic fluid level during pregancy is that it acts as a barometer of how the baby is doing. Too much fluid (polyhydramnios) or too little fluid (oligohydramnios) can mean that the pregnancy is in some difficulty. Amniotic fluid is constantly being produced during the pregnancy. Large amounts of fluid are exchanged between the mother and the fetus and the amniotic fluid and the fetus. The reason that amniotic fluid is sampled for chromosome analysis is that amniotic fluid holds live fetal cells that are sloughed off, or urinated or breathed into the amniotic fluid by the fetus and these cells can be grown and analyzed. It is like performing a needle biopsy on the fetus without ever touching the fetus. At birth, if we wanted to study the chromosomes of the baby we would have to remove blood from the baby to be tested. During pregnancy, the amniotic fluid can play the same role without disturbing the fetus through physical manipulation.

f. How much fluid is removed and why?

When amniocentesis is performed between 11 and 14 weeks gestation 6-10 cc's of fluid is removed; between 14.1 weeks and 23 weeks gestation 10-16 cc's of fluid is removed. When the procedure is performed, the extracted amniotic fluid is placed in (2 to 3 sterile vials) between 11 and 14 weeks and (3 to 4 vials) between 14.1 and 23 weeks. The reason for this is:

1. Separating the fluid helps prevent contamination and allows each of the specimens to be cultured to lower the likelihood that cells will not grow.
2. When the laboratory sets up a specimen for chromosome analysis, it sets up an A specimen (vial 1), a B specimen (vial 2), a C specimen (vial 3) and an amniotic fluid AFP (vial 3 or 4). This depends on how much fluid is obtained and weeks gestation.
3. Different tests can be performed on the different vials.
4. During the chromosome analysis cells must constantly be maintained and grown until a case is considered finished by the laboratory. This is usually about 14 days following the procedure. If any additional tests (i.e. DNA, metabolic tests) are required then the amniocytes (baby's cells from the amniotic fluid) will have to be maintained until the special tests have been completed. If the cells are not maintained then an amniocentesis may have to be repeated to get more fetal cells to be tested. Most women agree that one amniocentesis per pregnancy is enough.
5. If an abnormal result is found in the lab, it can be confirmed by examining the other sterile vials.
6. A laboratory diagnosis is ideally confirmed by observing the result in at least two of the specimens yielding the same chromosome result. For normal cases two specimens are studied. In abnormal results usually all three specimens are reviewed to confirm the diagnosis.
7. After 14.1 weeks approximately 2 cc's of the specimen will be reserved to perform an amniotic fluid AFP.
8. Some of the specimen is usually frozen for 6-12 months. This may be used to confirm the original diagnosis if necessary, after the baby is born.

g. How long does it take for amniotic fluid to be replaced?

The amniotic fluid usually replaces itself in less than 12-24 hours after the procedure. When the volume of amniotic fluid drops additional fluid is produced. The fluid is exchanged every 12-24 hours which keeps the fluid clean for the fetus.

h. Will the amnio hurt?

This question is the most frequently asked question. It is asked more often than the risk for miscarriage after CVS, early amniocentesis and amniocentesis. For the transabdominal amniocentesis most doctors will numb the skin of the abdomen with local anesthesia. Some doctors take a small needle and anesthetize under the skin where the needle will be inserted during the procedure. Most patients will feel very little. A few women might feel a slight itching or stinging sensation when the amniotic fluid is removed. This sensation is temporary and usually goes away once the needle is removed. Doctors who perform amnio will always try to stick the patient a single time with the needle.

Some of our friends who have had amniocentesis actually felt that the procedure was easier and less traumatic than when they had blood taken. We doubt that every woman would agree with this. We believe that if the amniotic fluid could be removed by osmosis that 100% of the women would choose to have it removed in this way.

The rule of thumb is that the lower on the abdomen that the procedure has to be performed, the more sensitive it will be for the patient. There appears to be more pain receptors in this region, therefore there is a greater chance of feeling the procedure. The whole procedure, from start to finish, usually takes less than 10 minutes. Most of this time is spent choosing the location for the procedure and sterile preparation of the site. Some women have complained that the most painful part of the procedure is having to have a full bladder (12-36 oz) for 45 minutes prior to the procedure.

Most of the discomfort, if any, is after the procedure has been completed. When the local anesthesia wears off, some women may experience some cramping and contractions. This is normal and usually ends in 12-24 hours after the procedure. Usually a small wash cloth or heating pad held over the site of the cramping can help relieve some of the pain. A small percentage of women (1%-2%) might have some bruising from the procedure at the needle insertion site. This, too, may be relieved by using a heating pad.

i. What is the difference between transabdominal amniocentesis and transvaginal amniocentesis?

Transabdominal amniocentesis means that the procedure is performed via the abdomen. Transvaginal amniocentesis means that the procedure is performed via the vagina. Virtually all amniocentesis that are performed today are performed via the abdomen route rather than via the vagina for a number of reasons: 1. Some doctors favor transabdominal amniocentesis because it poses less of a risk of introducing bacteria into the amniotic sac and causing infection of the fetus or amniotic fluid. 2. In order to perform transvaginal amniocentesis the doctor many times has to pass the needle through the bladder to reach the uterus. This procedure is extremely painful for the patient. 3. There is a slightly greater risk of miscarriage following a transvaginal amniocentesis versus a transabdominal amniocentesis.

j. What does amniocentesis screen for?

Amniocentesis screens for virtually all of the known chromosomal abnormalities that can be detected with today's technology. What that means is that the fetus has neither too many chromosomes, too few chromosomes or that parts of one chromosome have not broken and reattached with parts of other chromosomes. The amniotic fluid AFP test can help to detect small open neural tube or gastrointestinal wall defects that might not be seen with the ultrasound.

k. How long has amniocentesis been available?

Although amniocentesis was being performed in the late 1960's to the early 1970's, the procedure was considered experimental. In the late 1970's a study comparing women who did and did not have amniocentesis showed only a slightly higher risk (1:200 to 1:500) for miscarriage following the procedure.

l. Can any harm come to the fetus or the mother during the amniocentesis?

The greatest risk to the mother is a possible infection from the procedure. As with all surgical procedures, care is taken to keep the site of the procedure totally sterile. The risk for infection following the procedure is very small. The other risk to the mother is the possibility of premature rupture of membranes or miscarriage following the procedure. This happens in approximately 5 out of 400 procedures performed and compares with an approximate miscarriage risk of 4 in 400 even if amniocentesis is not performed. The greatest risk to the fetus is injury to the fetus or umbilical cord by the needle during the procedure. This risk can be lowered by using ultrasound guidance to view the needle in relationship to the fetus before, during and after the procedure. There is always of risk that the procedure can trigger a miscarriage or premature rupture of membranes. Warning signs include a loss of amniotic fluid, cramping or bleeding. If the mother sees any of these warning signs, she should contact her doctor. Most of the symptoms disappear in hours or days and the pregnancy will usually proceed to term.

m. Is Down syndrome the only thing that amniocentesis screens for?

Amniocentesis can help rule out almost all of the known chromosomal abnormalities in the fetus. Down syndrome is one of more than 100 named chromosomal syndromes or abnormalities that are screened for. There are many other chromosomal abnormalities that can be identified with amniocentesis but are not specifically named. The interpretation of chromosomes has continued to evolve over many years. Current techniques are highly reliable in identifying almost all of the major chromosomal abnormalities thus far described. Ongoing work continues to identify conditions previously unidentified. The karyotype demonstrates the chromosomes of the fetus. In every cell of every "normal" human being there should be 46 chromosomes; 22 pairs of chromosomes called autosomes, numbered 1-22 and two sex chromosomes. In a "normal" fetus, half of the chromosomes come from the mother and half from the father. A normal male karyotype is 46,XY and a normal female karyotype is 46,XX. A karyotype that has a greater number of chromosomes (i.e. Down syndrome 47,XX,+21 or 47,XY,+21) or a fewer number of chromosomes (i.e. Turner syndrome 45,XO) is considered to be an abnormal karyotype. Depending on the karyotype, the individual may or may not demonstrate identifiable abnormalities. When a laboratory says that the fetus' chromosomes are normal, it means that the number of chromosomes is 46, the sex of the chromosomes are appropriately male or female and neither extra chromosomal material or missing chromosomal material was identified. Also, parts of chromosomes have not been exchanged.

n. How active can I be after the amnio?

There is no right or wrong answer to this question. It really is up to the individual. Physicians ideally would like to see you diminish your activity (heavy lifting, sports) for the first 24-48 hours after the procedure to be aware of any subtle changes that might occur. One patient rode her bike to the procedure and then rode her bike home with no ill affects. Another patient had her procedure and ran a 5K the next day also with no ill affect. A third patient participated in a horse race the day of the procedure, again with no ill affect. Although these examples represent extremes, it helps demonstrate that different women respond differently to the procedure.

o. How long is the needle?

The needle is 3 1/2 inches long and can reach the uterus in virtually every patient. The needle itself only goes in about 1 1/2 to 2 inches.

p. What type of anesthesia is used?

Local anesthesia is used to numb the skin and outer surface of the uterus. Lidocaine (xylocaine) is chosen because it acts almost immediately and its effects last less than 20 minutes. It contains no epinephrine (that part of the anesthetic that can cause an anxious feeling or rapid heart rate when given by a dentist). It has no known adverse affects on the fetus.

q. How long does the amniocentesis take to perform? What about for twins and triplets?

The actual amniocentesis procedure take less than 10 minutes per fetus, so twins would take 20 minutes and triplets would take 30 minutes. Some programs perform a targeted Level II ultrasound to study the development of the fetus and the integrity of the pregnancy prior to performing the procedure. Each ultrasound study takes 30-45 minutes per fetus. The entire procedure takes about one hour per fetus, 1 1/2 to 2 hours for two fetuses and 2 1/2 to 3 hours for three fetuses. The three ultrasound studies are performed and the amniocentesis is performed on all three fetuses sequentially at the very end of the ultrasound study. The needle is in the abdomen for only a matter of minutes even if multiple fetuses are being studied.

r. How long does it take for amnio cells to grow and be analyzed by the lab?

Amniotic fluid chromosome results will usually be reported in 8-10 days following the procedure. Occassionally, it can take up to 14-15 days to get a result. This does NOT mean that anything is wrong with your baby. Most labs check all specimens on day six or seven following the procedure to determine if an early diagnosis can be made. (Remember: Normal fetal cells grow at different rates).

s. How do you know that you have sampled each fetus in a multiple gestation pregnancy?

When amniotic fluid is removed from the first fetus' amniotic sac, a safe vegetable dye is introduced into the amniotic fluid so that it can be distinguished from the non-tested amniotic sac of the second fetus. If fluid is removed and contains dye, the same sac was entered a second time.

t. Do you have to be stuck twice for twins?

This will depend upon the relationship between the two amniotic sacs. If one sac lies above the other, it may be possible to remove the fluid from the lower twin, insert dye, and then without removing the needle, raise the needle and remove the amniotic fluid from the second fetus. More often then not the sacs are next to each other, and a second stick of the needle will have to be done to reach the second sac. Most physicians who perform amniocentesis try to limit the number of times that they have to stick the patient with the needle.

u. Does the procedure ever need to be repeated?

An amniocentesis may have to be repeated for the following reasons:

1. The amniotic fluid fails to grow cells that can be analyzed.
2. Not enough cells are removed at the time of the procedure. Maternal blood contamination of the specimen may delay or prevent growth of cells.
3. The mother has a contraction that reduces the pool of fluid in the chosen site.
4. The mother or father who are given an "abnormal" chromosome result may request a second amniocentesis so that they can confirm the diagnosis.
5. Results are inconclusive or confusing.

The need for repeat amniocentesis occurs less than 1 in 100 cases.

v. Is being tender after the amniocentesis normal?

Yes. Anytime that you put a needle in a muscle (and the uterus is a big muscle) you may get some cramping. In a few cases, the amniocentesis will cause minor contractions and possible bruising of the area where the procedure was performed. All of these symptoms should go away in 12-24 hours after the procedure and can be minimized by applying a heating pad to the tender area.

w. What is amniocentesis for fetal lung maturity and when is it performed?

Amniocentesis to determine fetal lung maturity is a non-genetic procedure performed by a physician in the hospital to determine whether the lungs of the baby are mature enough to survive outside the uterus. This procedure is usually performed after 31 weeks gestation and can be repeated up until delivery. This test is usually performed by the hospital lab where you will deliver or at an outside laboratory. It is not usually performed by a genetics laboratory. Chromosome studies of the fetus are usually not performed. If you want genetic studies performed on the amniotic fluid, you must request it at the time of the procedure.

AMNIOTIC BANDS

a. What is an amniotic band and how, when and why does it occur?

During the pregnancy, as the fetus develops, the room available for the fetus inside the uterus becomes more compact. Even though the uterus is a very stretchable muscle and can usually accommodate single or multiple pregnancies up to 9 to 9 1/2 months gestation, a very small percentage of pregnancies have amniotic bands occur. Amniotic bands occur when an area of the amniotic sac (sac that encapsulates and protects the fetus) loses its integrity. The amniotic sac should grow as the fetus grows but sometimes bands may form which may attach to the fetus leading to constriction of normal organs.

The cause of the amniotic band in the uterus is not absolutely known. Leakage of small amounts of fluid from the amniotic sac surrounding the baby, an infection during the pregnancy or rupture of membranes in pregnancy is known to cause the formation of amniotic fluid bands. It is believed that amniotic fluid bands can occur late in the first trimester, during the second trimester and can occur but is much less likely in the third trimester.

The amniotic band is usually identified after a malformation is identified in the fetus or newborn infant. Since amniotic bands usually occur due to amniotic fluid leakage, it usually does not repeat in subsequent pregnancies. The occurrence of an amniotic bandlike syndrome in more than one infant by the same mother should prompt an investigation for a possible reason for the event. In some of these patients a dye study of the non-pregnant uterus (hysterosalpingogram - usually a minor surgical procedure which requires only a short stay of several hours in the hospital) will show scars in the uterus. If these scars are identified, they should be removed surgically.

An amniotic band syndrome found a second time in the same mother is usually not due to a family disorder or syndrome since the fetal position during each pregnancy varies. Recurrent amniotic band abnormalities that manifest themselves will very likely be in different positions depending upon the fetal position. When this has occurred in a previous pregnancy, and the scars are removed surgically, it is prudent to suggest serial ultrasound studies throughout the pregnancy to identify and montior amniotic bands in relationship to the fetus. Even if a mother experiences an amniotic band in one pregnancy, the risk for subsequent recurrence is very low.

BETA HCG - SERUM HUMAN CHORIONIC GONADOTROPIN (HCG)

a. What is the difference between HCG values in early pregnancy and HCG in AFP3?

The early pregnancy test is called urine beta HCG which is a specific test for the hormone beta HCG used to identify pregnant women. A false positive beta HCG and a false negative can occur if the test is run too early (i.e. if ovulation did not occur until later than the expected time of a woman's cycle). Beta HCG studies performed on maternal blood early in pregnancy can help identify whether a woman is pregnant or not. Maternal serum HCG (MSHCG) is a test performed on a mother's blood, not urine. This test is usually performed between 15 and 20 weeks gestation.

The beta HCG in AFP3 is used to help identify a fetus that is at a greater risk for Down syndrome. MSHCG is part of AFP3 - The Triple Screen (AFP, Beta HCG and Estriol) and can assist in the detection of up to 89% of Down syndrome fetuses which women over the age of 35 years may be carrying, and 55%-66% in women under the age of 35.

1. MSHCG levels tend to be high in pregnancies with trisomy 21 fetuses, some trisomy 13 and some trisomy 18 fetuses.
2. MSHCG levels have also been shown to be low in some cases of trisomy 18 fetuses.
3. MSHCG has also been found to be elevated in abdominal wall defects.

b. If my HCG value doubles every 2nd or 3rd day early in pregnancy, is that normal? If not, why?

Yes, the beta HCG values should double every 2nd or 3rd day in a normal pregnancy. Maternal blood testing for beta HCG can be used in the early first trimester to provide information as to whether the pregnancy is proceeding normally or whether the pregnancy will possibly result in a miscarriage or tubal pregnancy (a pregnancy in the fallopian tube rather than in the uterus). Low HCG values or failure to follow this trend of doubling are associated with a greater likelihood of miscarriage or tubal pregnancy.

BLOOD CHROMOSOMES

a. What are blood chromosomes?

Blood chromosomes studies are performed on cells that are cultured from the blood of a patient. By growing the white blood cells of the patient and studying the cells when they are dividing a determination can be made whether the chromosomes are normal or abnormal. This study can be performed on umbilical cord blood, blood from a newborn, a child or an adult. Usually, a small amount of blood (3-5 cc's) in a heparinzed (non-clotting) tube is required.

b. When and why are blood chromosomes studied?

Umbilical cord blood sampling is sometimes performed after an abnormal result from CVS, early amniocentesis, or amniocentesis to confirm the diagnosis. A newborn who was not offered prenatal diagnosis but is having medical complications and/or has multiple congenital anomalies or abnormalities that indicate possible chromosomal syndromy will have blood drawn to confirm or rule out an abnormality. This diagnosis can help the health care professional decide how aggressive to be with lifesaving techniques on the baby.

An adult may have blood chromosomes for any of the following reasons:

1. As part of paternity testing to confirm or rule out whether the man is the biological parent of the child.

2. A history of multiple miscarriages (two or more consecutive losses) to rule out a chromosomal abnormality in either parent. Some studies have shown that as many as 13% of couples that have two or more consecutive miscarriages have been associated with a chromosomal abnormality, usually a translocation (where parts of two chromosomes break off and exchange with one another) in one or both parents.

3. A physical exam by a health care professional suggests a chromosomal abnormality or syndrome.

4. A pregnant couple gets an abnormal chromosome result from a karyotype study performed on their fetus which is not known to be associated with a definitive problem. Both parents would be offered blood chromosomes to rule out a chromosomal abnormality in one parent. If either parent has the same abnormality as the child and is otherwise normal then it is likely that the fetus will also be normal. (See Blood Chromosome Figures #1, #2, #3 p. 47-49.)

5. Women who have never been able to conceive particularly if they have abnormalities of their sexual organs or menstrual pattern. Blood chromosomes help to rule out Turner syndrome (45,XO) where one X chromosome is missing or other sex chromosomal abnormalities.

6. For families that have a history of certain cancers, particularly leukemia or lymphoma, blood chromosome studies might be performed serially to confirm the diagnosis, to help follow the course of the disease, the effectiveness of chemotherapy and the likelihood of recurrence of the cancer. This is very experimental at the publication of this book.

CHROMOSOMAL ABNORMALITIES

a. What is a karyotype?

The karyotype demonstrates chromosomes of an individual. In each cell of every genetically "normal" human being there are 46 chromosomes composed of 22 pairs of chromosomes (called autosomes) numbered 1-22 and two sex chromosomes. These chromosomes are first viewed in a metaphase (See Metaphase Figure #4) and then cut up and matched into pairs. They are then placed on a karyotype grid sheet (See Karyotype Record Figure #5). In a normal baby, half of the chromosomes come from the biological mother and half from the biological father. A normal male karyotype is 46,XY and a normal female karyotype is 46,XX.

Any karyotype that has a greater number of chromosomes than 46 (i.e. Down syndrome 47,XX,+21 or 47,XY,+21) or less than 46 (i.e. Turner syndrome 45,XO) is considered an abnormal karyotype. The individual may or may not demonstrate identifiable abnormalities. When a lab says that a karyotype is "normal" it means that the number of chromosomes is 46, the sex of the chromosomes are appropriately male or female and no extra or missing chromosomal material was identified, nor have parts of chromosomes been exchanged.

b. What is a normal male and/or female karyotype?

A normal male karyotype is 46,XY (See Male Karyotype Figure #6) and a normal female karyotype is 46,XX (See Female Karyotype Figure #7).

c. What is Down syndrome?

Down syndrome or trisomy 21 is a condition in which a third chromosome #21 is introduced into a basically normal karyotype (See Down syndrome Figure #8). Babies with trisomy 21 used to be called "Mongoloid" due to their almond shaped eyes and faces. The name has been changed to trisomy 21 or Down syndrome to remove the possible racial connotation associated with the term Mongoloid. Among the general population Down syndrome is believed to be the most common genetic abnormality. However, in the genetics labs across the country sex chromosomal abnormalities are seen more often than Down syndrome. Down syndrome babies are usually identified by the following characteristics:

1. Poor body tone.
2. Flat faces.
3. Eyes which slant downward.
4. Large tongue.
5. Decreased IQ (average 52).
6. Mental retardation.
7. Heart defects (approximately 40% of infants).

d. What is Turner syndrome?

Turner syndrome describes an individual who has a karyotype of 45,XO and occurs when a female child does not inherit a second X chromosome from either parent, or the X is not replicated when the cell divides (See Turner Syndrome Figure #9). From a genetics standpoint these patients are female but are missing the second X that makes them a "normal" female. Women who have never been able to conceive, have had few or no periods since puberty could possibly have Turner syndrome. Other characteristics for Turner syndrome are:

1. Short stature.
2. Short neck or "webbed" neck.
3. Broad chest with widely spaced nipples.
4. "Puffy" hands or feet.
5. Heart defects (approximately 20%).
6. Mean IQ is normal (approximately 95).

e. What is a translocation?

A translocation describes a karyotype where part of a chromosome or chromosomes break off and reattach to other chromosomes (See Translocation Figure #10). When a translocation is found in the fetus, blood chromosome studies of both parents is usually recommended to rule out that the translocation was inherited from either parent. The prognosis for babies with translocations is better if the translocation is inherited from either or both parents rather than a new chromosomal translocation.

f. What is mosaicism?

Mosaicism means that an individual or fetus demonstrates more than one cell type, each with a different chromosome complement. There are usually normal cells and a percentage of abnormal cells (See Mosaic Chromosome Report Figure #11). This ratio of normal to abnormal cells can be measured and will be recorded by the lab. This is done by counting the percentage of normal to abnormal cells (e.g 90:10, 50:50, 10:90 normal to abnormal cells respectively). Two or more karyotypes will be made for the fetus with a mosaic result; one normal karyotype, and one or more representing the abnormal karyotypes. The progosis for fetuses with both normal and abnormal cells is usually better than for fetuses in which every cell in the body has the chromosomal abnormality.

CHORIONIC VILLUS SAMPLING (CVS)

a. What is CVS, what does it screen for, and when can you do it?

Transabdominal amniocentesis has been the standard method for obtaining amniotic fluid and/or fetal cells for prenatal diagnostic testing. Amniocentesis is usually performed between 15-18 weeks gestation. The desirability of performing the procedure earlier in pregnancy is obvious. The earlier you get the information, the earlier you can make decisions regarding the pregnancy. Sampling can be accomplished by taking cells from the chorion frondosum (chorion = membrane encircling the fetus and frondosum (shaggy) = the portion of the chorion where villi (a projection from the surface) persist forming the fetal part of the placenta. Chorionic villi can be obtained fairly early in pregnancy (9-11 weeks from the first day of the last menstrual period) and usually have the same chromosomes as the fetus. Therefore, many of the diseases tested for by amniocentesis can be detected earlier with chorionic villus sampling.

Retrieval of the chorionic villi was initially performed by

placing instruments through the vagina and cervix into the uterus. Recently, procedures have been described to obtain chorionic villus tissue by placing a needle through the abdomen into the placenta and aspirating villus tissue into a syringe prepared with a solution used to grow cells. By using a transabdominal method for chorionic villus sampling the small risk of an intrauterine infection by the vaginal method can be avoided. Most studies show no difference in the risk from either procedure.

b. What is the difference between CVS and amniocentesis?

1. The risk of miscarriage following CVS is slightly higher (1%-2%) than amniocentesis (1%) and the accuracy of the test results is slightly lower for CVS (98%-99%) than amniocentesis (99%).
2. If CVS is performed and the fetus is female, it may not be possible to rule out that maternal contamination of the specimen occurred and that the result is the mother's karyotype rather than the fetus. If the karyotype is male then maternal contamination can be ruled out.
3. There is a 1%-2% chance that a CVS with a female karyotype will have to be repeated with an amniocentesis at 15-18 weeks to confirm the chromosomal results.
4. An amniotic fluid AFP can not be performed on a CVS specimen because the procedure is performed too early in pregnancy.
5. A fetal evaluation by ultrasound can not be done at the time of the CVS (9-11 weeks gestation). Therefore, the following procedures should be considered.

   a. Maternal serum alphafetoprotein or AFP3 should be done at 15-20 weeks to help rule out an open neural tube defect or abdominal wall defect.
   b. A Level II (targeted ultrasound of the fetus) should be done at 15-17 weeks to evaluate the fetus. If the CVS showed a female karyotype, the ultrasound should also be used to confirm the sex of the fetus.

Since the CVS is performed on placental cells rather than on the amniotic fluid cells, all labs will qualify their results by saying that there is always a chance of maternal contamination. By 11 weeks the amniotic fluid begins to appear. Many women who might have chosen CVS to get an early diagnosis might choose early amniocentesis because a female karyotype following amniocentesis is more likely to represent the fetal karyotype.

c. Are there limb abnormalities associated with CVS?

Recently, the media alerted the public to a possible relationship between CVS and birth defects. Specifically, a few centers in the United Kingdom and the United States reported unusual limb defects and/or facial defects which were reported in a greater number of infants whose mothers had undergone CVS than might otherwise be expected.

It has been somewhat confusing even for health care professionals to sort through this information. Some centers have temporarily abandoned the procedure. Advocates of CVS have suggested that the timing of the procedure, the amount of tissue removed to be sampled, and the expertise of the physician performing the procedure might be the most important factors behind the limb abnormalities. One study had 4:400 babies that had limb and/or facial abnormalities following the CVS. A more recent study suggested a risk of 5 in 10,000 procedures. These same abnormalities to date **have not** been noted in early amniocentesis and amniocentesis.

d. Is the miscarriage risk following CVS higher than amniocentesis?

Since miscarriage occurs more frequently early in pregnancy, more miscarriages occur following CVS than amniocentesis. Miscarriage rates for CVS may be as high as 6%-8%. It is estimated that the increased risk for miscarriage attributed to the procedure itself is no higher than 1%-2%. As with amniocentesis; infection, hemorrhage and/or spontaneous rupture of the membranes (bag of water) or premature labor can occur.

e. Do I have to have an amniocentesis repeated at 15-18 weeks if the karyotype from CVS is female?

Since chromosomes from CVS (which is really a placental biopsy) may NOT represent the fetus in all cases, a follow-up amniocentesis may be recommended to confirm the findings of

CVS studies (approximately 1%-2%). It may not always be possible to know that the chromosomes studied do represent the fetus. A follow-up ultrasound is recommended at 15-17 weeks gestation to monitor the progress of the pregnancy, the fetal structural integrity and confirm the sex of the fetus. If a possible discrepancy is detected, an amniocentesis would be recommended. Chorionic villus sampling is performed too early to allow diagnosis of 85%-90% of open spinal defects (e.g. spina bifida) or abdominal wall defects that can be diagnosed with ultrasound and amniocentesis.

DNA Testing

a. What else can be tested for before or during the pregnancy?

Most metabolic disorders are inherited in an autosomal recessive manner. Both parents would have to be gene carriers of the abnormality and each parent would have to pass the affected gene on to the baby for the baby to be affected. Carrier testing may be available to determine if one or both parents have one or more abnormal genes.

Some diseases are carried on the X chromosome (X-linked). Since males have only one X, they demonstrate the disease. Females have two X chromosomes. In most (but not all) cases females are usually carriers and are not affected. 50% of their male children would be affected and 50% of their female children would be carriers.

The following list is a compilation of DNA or special laboratory tests that were available at the time of the publication of this book. Remember, that if there is a particular disease that affects your family but is not on the list, then you need to contact your health care professional and see if the testing has become available.

ALPHA-1-ANTITRYPSIN DEFICIENCY:

A cause of liver disease or lung disease or immune problems.

ANGELMAN SYNDROME:

A specific type of severe mental retardation. May appear as a "happy puppet" meaning that the patient acts like a puppet.

ASHKENAZIC GENETIC DISEASE (TAY-SACHS, GAUCH-ERS, CYSTIC FIBROSIS):

Specific metabolic diseases. Autosomal recessive.

BECKER MUSCULAR DYSTROPHY:

A type of progressive muscular deterioration which is similar but milder than Duchenne Muscular Dystrophy.

CHARCOT-MARIE-TOOTH:

Nerve-muscle degeneration disease. Can be inherited in an autosomal dominant or autosomal recessive manner.

CITRULLINEMIA:

Metabolic disease. Autosomal recessive.

CONGENITAL ADRENAL HYPERPLASIA(21-HYDROXY-LASE DEFICIENCY):

There are various forms of this disease ranging from mild to very severe. The most mild demonstrates ambiguous genitalia (there is an inability to be able to distinguish whether the genitalia are male or female) to the most severe form involving convulsions and sometimes even death. Autosomal recessive.

CRI-DU-CHAT "Cry of the Cat":

Mental retardation, small head, cat-like cry due to a missing piece of the top of chromosome #5.

CYSTIC FIBROSIS (CF):

Metabolic disease. Autosomal recessive.

DUCHENNE MUSCULAR DYSTROPHY:

Progressive muscle wasting disease, usually resulting in death before age 20. Affects males; females can be carriers. X-linked inheritance.

FACTOR VIII (AHG) - ANTI-HEMOPHILIAC GLOBULIN DEFICIENCY (HEMOPHILIA):

Blood factor which plays a role in the clotting of blood.

FACTOR IX (CHRISTMAS FACTOR DEFICIENCY):

Blood factor which plays a role in the clotting of blood.

FACTOR XIII:

Blood factor which plays a role in the clotting of blood.

FLUORESCENT IN-SITU HYBRIDIZATION:

Use of special stains to identify specific chromosomes or pieces of chromosomes.

FRAGILE-X SYNDROME:

Mental retardation in males, identified by a tendency of a small piece near the bottom of the X chromosome which seems to separate from the rest of the X chromosome under special culture conditions.

HIGH RESOLUTION CHROMOSOMES:

Examining chromosomes which have been specially treated to identify very small losses or gains of pieces of chromosomal material.

HUNTINGTON'S CHOREA:

Progressive brain deterioration which may not present until the 30's, 40's or 50's. Autosomal Dominant.

HURLER'S SYNDROME:

Metabolic disease. Autosomal recessive.

HURLER-SCHEIE DISEASE:

Metabolic disease. Autosomal dominant.

KENNEDY DISEASE:

Muscle wasting disease. X-linked inheritance.

LESCH-NYHAN DISEASE:

Metabolic disease. X-linked inheritance.

LOU GEHRIG'S DISEASE:

Also known as Amyotrophic Lateral Sclerosis (ALS). Muscle wasting disease. Both autosomal dominant and autosomal recessive inheritance has been described.

MEDIUM CHAIN ACYL-CoA DEHYROGENASE (MCAD):

Metabolic disease. Autosomal recessive.

MILLER-DIEKER:

Incomplete brain development often associated with an abnormality in the upper half of chromosome #17.

MYOTONIC DYSTROPHY:

Muscle disease. Autosomal dominant.

NEUROFIBROMATOSIS:

Development of benign or occassionally malignant tumors along the course of the nerves with occassional seizures. Multiple skin lesions (cafe-au lait spots) are present. Autosomal dominant.

NORRIE'S DISEASE:

Metabolic disease. Blindness, possible deafness or possible developmental delay. X-linked inheritance.

ORNITHINE TRANSCARBAMYLASE:

Metabolic disease. X-linked inheritance.

PATERNITY STUDIES - AMNIOTIC FLUID:

Retrieval and use of fetal cells suspended in the amniotic fluid to compare with a mother's white blood cells and those of a presumed father to determine paternity.

PHENYLKETONURIA (PKU):

Metabolic disease. Autosomal recessive.

POLYCYSTIC KIDNEY DISEASE:

Presence of many and/or large cysts in one or both kidneys and/or liver. Autosomal dominant and autosomal recessive inheritance have been described.

PRADER-WILLI:

A condition of developmental delay and compulsive overeating leading to obesity. A chromosomal abnormality may be present.

PROPRIONIC CoA:

Metabolic disease. Autosomal recessive.

RETINOBLASTOMA:

Development of a cancer in the back of the eye. Autosomal recessive.

SICKLE CELL DISEASE (BLACK ANCESTRY):

Blood disease causing anemia and blood clotting. Autosomal recessive.

TAY SACHS DISEASE (JEWISH/FRENCH CANADIAN ANCESTRY):

Fatal metabolic blood disease. Autosomal recessive.

THALASSEMIA (ITALIAN/ASIAN ANCESTRY):

Most common blood disease in caucasian populations. Increased occurence in Asians. Autosomal recessive.

WOLF-HIRSCHORN:

Growth and mental retardation, small head, "Greek warrior helmet" appearing face, cleft lips and/or cleft palate and/or heart defects. A small piece of the short arm of chromosome #4 is usually absent.

———————————

Some of these tests listed above can only be performed on the mother and/or father of the baby, but not on amniocytes (baby's amniotic fluid cells). Some of these tests are more reliable if performed on the child after he/she is born, but many parents think that it is too late to find out about a problem after the delivery. The information from these tests may tell you if the fetus or patient is:

1. Affected with a disease of trait.
2. A carrier of the disease or trait.
3. Free from acquiring the disease or trait.

DOWN SYNDROME

a. What is a Down syndrome risk?

In the last 2-5 years there have been many tests introduced to help detect pregnancies that might be at an increased risk for possible problems. The major indication for prenatal diagnosis since 1972 is a maternal age related risk for a 35 year old woman for having a child with Down syndrome. These children have three chromosome 21's instead of the normal two. The maternal age risk for a 35 year old woman for having a child with Down syndrome is 1:270. The reason that women over the age of 35 are routinely offered prenatal diagnosis by genetic amniocentesis is the fact that these women have a greater risk for having a child with a chromosomal abnormality than the risk for miscarriage following the procedure.

Although, most Down syndrome babies are born to women under the age of 35, this group has not traditionally been offered prenatal diagnosis. Greater attempts to help diagnose infants with Down Syndrome or other chromosomal abnormalities have been directed towards women less than 35 years old. The triple screen or AFP3 was introduced to help identify women at increased risk. Women who are offered this testing will be given a Down syndrome risk that will be less than, equal to or greater than the risk for a 35 year old woman (1:270). Some labs are using 1:190, some labs are using 1:200, most labs are using 1:270 and one lab is using 1:384 (the risk for a 30 year old) as a cutoff. Needless to say, your test result could be normal or abnormal depending upon the lab that is chosen to run the AFP or the AFP3. Any woman who has a calculated risk greater than or equal to 1:270 will be offered prenatal diagnosis by genetic amniocentesis. Remember, if your test result comes back greater than 1:270 it does not mean that your baby has Down syndrome. It simply means that you and your health care professional should consider testing to rule out possible Down syndrome.

b. Do CVS, early amniocentesis and amniocentesis all identify Down syndrome?

Yes. CVS can identify Down syndrome as early as 9-11 weeks gestation, early amniocentesis from 11-14 weeks and amniocentesis from 15-23 weeks. When a sample is received by a lab, the specimen is tested for chromosomal composition including Down syndrome or any extra or missing chromosomal material that can be identified.

c. Does AFP/AFP2/AFP3 detect Down syndrome?

No. All three serum blood tests are screening tests to help identify pregnancies that **might** be at an increased risk for Down syndrome. This is a statistical risk rather than an accurate identification of Down syndrome. A positive AFP test for an increased risk for Down syndrome does not mean that the fetus has Down syndrome. It simply means that the pregnancy is at an increased risk and patients should be offered prenatal diagnosis by amniocentesis to rule out Down syndrome. A negative AFP, AFP2, or AFP3 test does not guarantee that your baby will not have Down syndrome. AFP3 can help identify up to 89% of Down syndrome babies but there are 11% of those babies that will be missed. Although, other chromosomal abnormalities are detected with AFP3, almost 50% of chromosomal abnormalities will be missed. Because of this, AFP3 blood screening is NOT currently believed to be a replacement for more definitive testing like CVS or amniocentesis in patients at increased risk.

d. Are all Down syndrome babies alike?

No. There are different gradations of Down syndrome. Babies with Down syndrome have similar physical features, however, IQ, mental retardation, speech, coordination and attitude vary from patient to patient. A 100% Down syndrome baby is one that has an extra 21 chromosome in every cell of his/her body. A mosaic Down syndrome baby has two or more cell lines with both normal and abnormal cells. This normal to abnormal cell ratio can be measured. The prognosis for an increased IQ in mosaic Down syndrome infants has been documented.

e. If the baby has Down syndrome can you predict the baby's IQ from prenatal diagnosis?

No. Although, we can tell the patient whether 100% of the baby's cells are affected or whether some normal cells are present, there is no current technology to evaluate IQ or mental retardation prenatally.

EARLY AMNIOCENTESIS

a. What is early amniocentesis, when can you do it, and what does it screen for?

Amniocentesis is the withdrawal of a sample of amniotic fluid from the bag of water surrounding the fetus. This fluid is usually obtained by introducing a needle through the abdomen and uterus after an ultrasound to choose the best and safest location. Some slight discomfort may be experienced when the needle is introduced. This procedure can be performed between 11 and 14 weeks gestation as long as there is enough amniotic fluid to safely sample. This test is slightly more reliable than CVS since fetal cells are suspended in the amniotic fluid. CVS is essentially a biopsy of the placenta. Usually (but not always) the chromosomes of the placenta and the fetus are the same. If a female karyotype is found on amniotic fluid, the chance for maternal contamination is almost zero. Early amniocentesis can screen for greater than 99% of the known chromosomal abnormalities. Like CVS, it can not screen for open neural tube defects or abdominal wall defects because it is done too early to perform an amniotic fluid AFP.

Ultrasound is performed to localize the placenta, to take measurements of the fetus, to look for some specific abnormalities and to determine whether more than one fetus is present. An occassional complication of the procedure is leakage of amniotic fluid which may be blood tinged, from the vagina after the procedure. The leakage is not considered a serious complication however, your health care professional should be notified. You may experience a few minor contractions following the procedure and should reduce your activities for the remainder of the day. As with all surgical procedures there is a possibility of infection. Every precaution is taken to prevent this.

In approximately two-thirds of patients, the placenta is located on the front of the uterus, towards your abdomen. In these cases it may be necessary to pass the needle through the placenta in order to obtain amniotic fluid. Most studies have shown that doing this does not increase the risk of early amniocentesis. Results from early amniocentesis depends on the growth of live cells contained in the amniotic fluid. Occassionally, (less than 1:100 amniocentesis) cells may fail to grow and it may be suggested that the procedure be repeated.

b. What is the miscarriage risk?

The risk of miscarriage from the early amniocentesis is low (less than 1:200 early amniocentesis procedures). In order to attempt to reduce the risk of miscarriage the procedure is usually performed under direct ultrasound guidance (watching the needle as it enters the uterus). The risks quoted were calculated when the procedure was not performed with ultrasound guidance. The actual risk for "early" amniocentesis versus amniocentesis at 15 weeks is unknown. It is known that a few more women miscarry when amniocentesis is performed prior to 15 weeks. Whether this slightly greater risk is due to the procedure or whether it would have occurred anyway is unknown. Some studies have suggested a slightly higher risk of injury to the fetus when the procedure is performed early. Other studies have not confirmed an increased risk.

ECTOPIC PREGNANCY

a. What is an ectopic pregnancy?

An "ectopic" pregnancy is defined as a pregnancy in any site outside of the uterine cavity. Although it usually refers to a pregnancy that implants in a fallopian tube, fertilized eggs can implant on the ovary, the intestines or other sites. These latter sites are very rare and very dangerous for the mother. The general populations risk for an ectopic pregnancy is 1:200 conceptions. However, this incidence may be rising due to sexually transmitted diseases. An ectopic pregnancy can occur in any patient.

b. What causes an ectopic pregnancy?

An ectopic pregnancy is caused by a fertilized egg that does not make it to the uterus to implant. The actual cause of why a fertilized egg implants in the fallopian tube versus the uterus is still unknown. Scarring of the fallopian tube, an abnormal or closed fallopian tube can help trap and allow the implantation of the fertilized egg.

c. How do you diagnose an ectopic pregnancy?

The diagnosis of an ectopic pregnancy/tubal pregnancy is still difficult. Usually a combination of maternal blood tests and ultrasound is necessary in order to diagnose the problem. Once an ectopic has been indentified, surgery by laparoscopic removal or opening the abdomen to remove the pregnancy are the most common approaches. Recently, some health care professionals have begun using a cancer drug called Methotrexate, which is either taken orally or injected directly into the pregnancy via the use of the laparoscope. Somewhere between 10%-20% of patients who have a drug trial for the ectopic as treatment will still require close supervision and surgery. The waiting period before attempting to conceive following an ectopic is two to three months. Consult your health care professional before engaging in sexual relations following an ectopic pregnancy.

d. Do I have a risk for recurrence of an ectopic pregnancy?

The recurrence risk for another tubal or ectopic pregnancy is approximately 10%-15%.

e. Am I at a greater risk for having an abnormal baby?

Although, once a patient has an ectopic or tubal pregnancy she is at a greater risk for recurrence of an ectopic pregnancy, there is no evidence that a family history of ectopic or tubal pregnancies increases the risk for a child with chromosomal or other abnormalities.

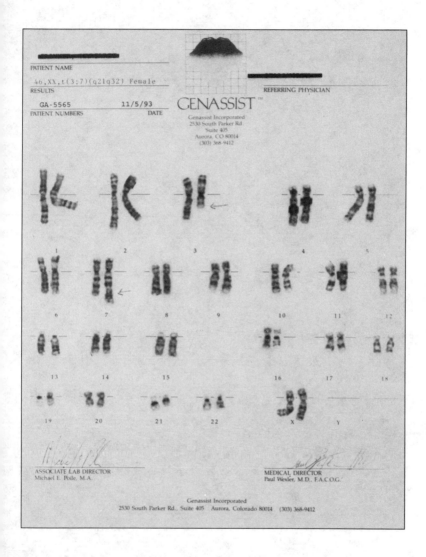

Figure 1 *Fetal cells from amniotic fluid showed chromosomal material exchanged between one chromosome #3 and one chromosome #7. (See arrows).*

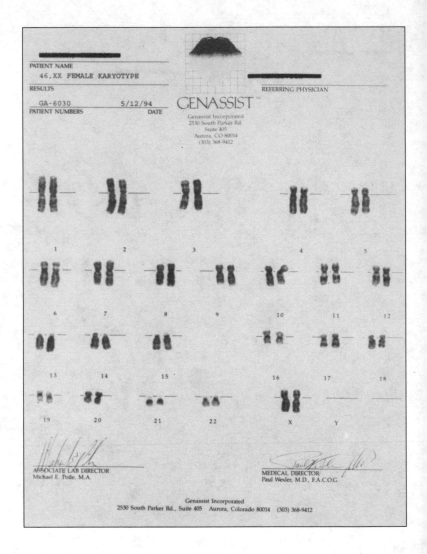

Figure 2 *Blood chromosome studies from the mother of the fetus shown in Figure 1. These chromosomes are normal.*

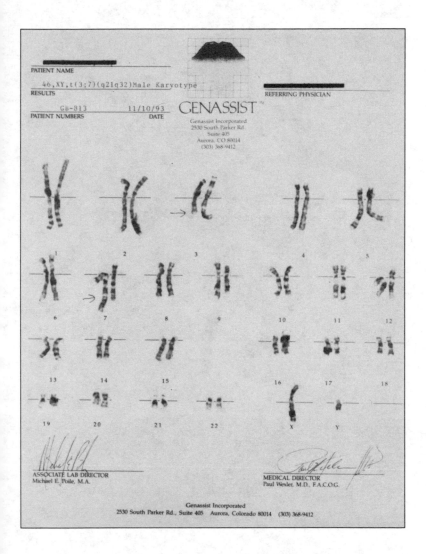

Figure 3 *Blood chromosome studies from the father of the fetus shown in Figure 1. A similar abnormality is seen. (See arrows).*

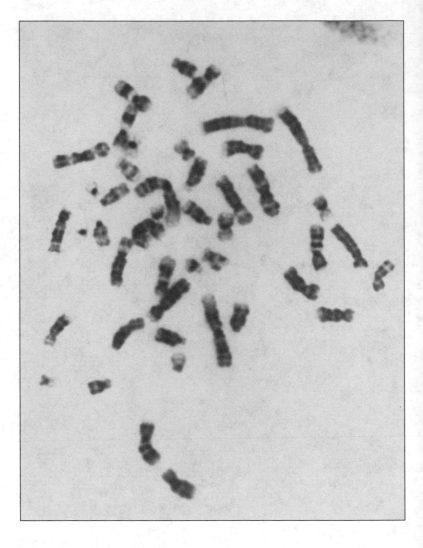

Figure 4 *Middle stage of cell division in which chromosomes are most easily studied.*

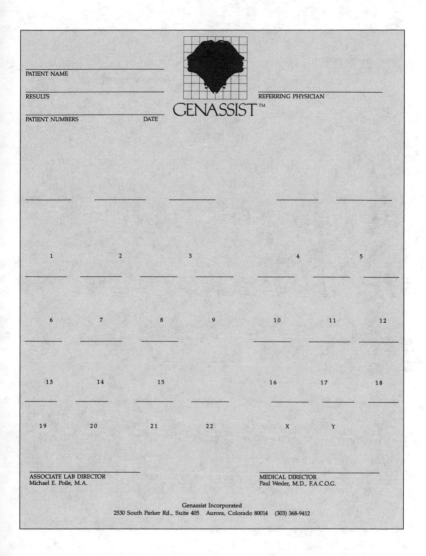

Figure 5 *"Grid" used for displaying matched chromosome pairs.*

52

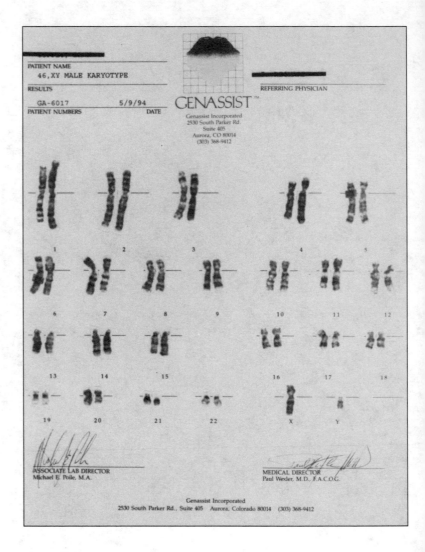

Figure 6 *Normal male karyotype, showing one X and one Y chromosome.*

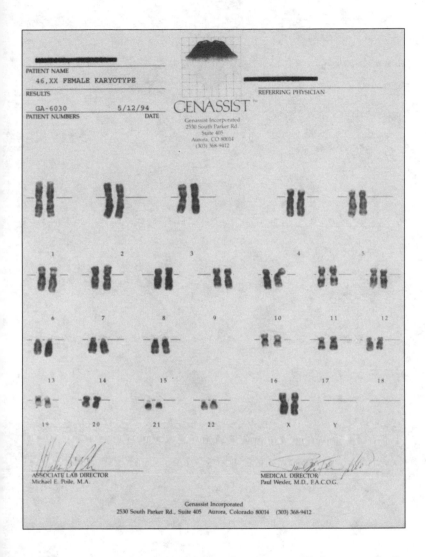

Figure 7 *Normal female karyotype, showing two X chromosomes. In females, no Y chromosome is present.*

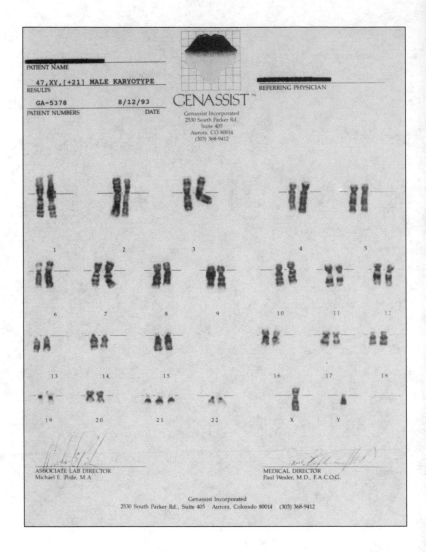

Figure 8 *Down syndrome karyotype. Note: three chromosomes above #21. This karyotype has 47 chromosomes rather than the normal 46.*

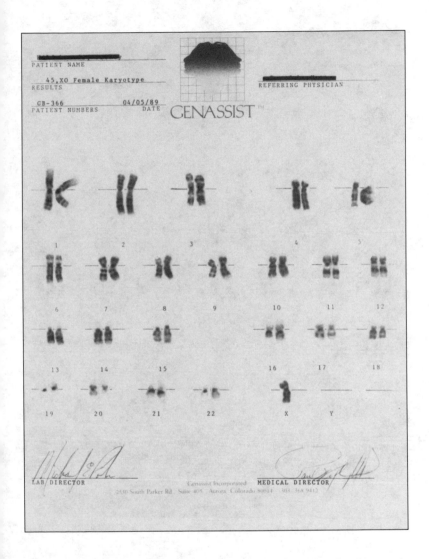

Figure 9 *Turner syndrome karyotype. Note: only one X chromosome is present. This karyotype has 45 chromosomes rather than the normal 46.*

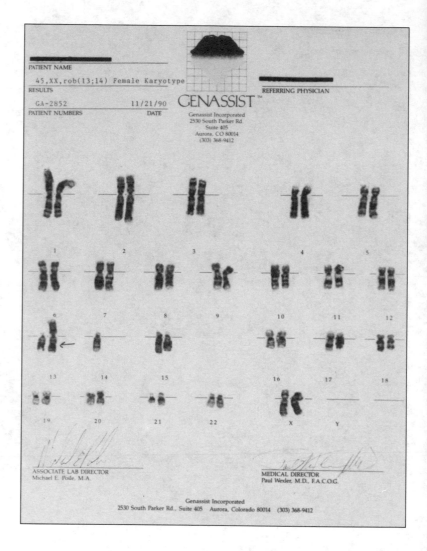

Figure 10 *Translocation between chromosome #13 and chromosome #14. One chromosome #14 has fused to the top of one chromosome #13.*

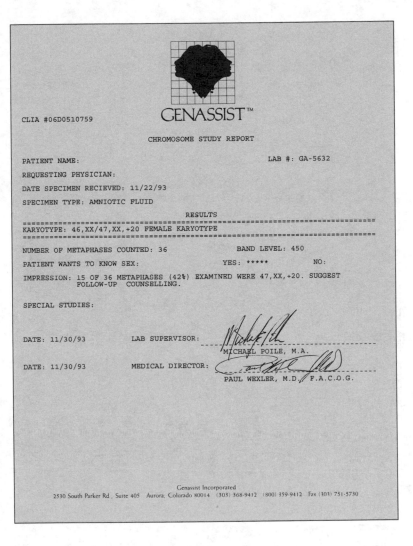

Figure 11 *"Mosaic" female karyotype. Some cells were normal having 46 chromosomes, including two X chromosomes. 42% of the cells had 47 chromosomes, including an extra chromosome #20.*

58

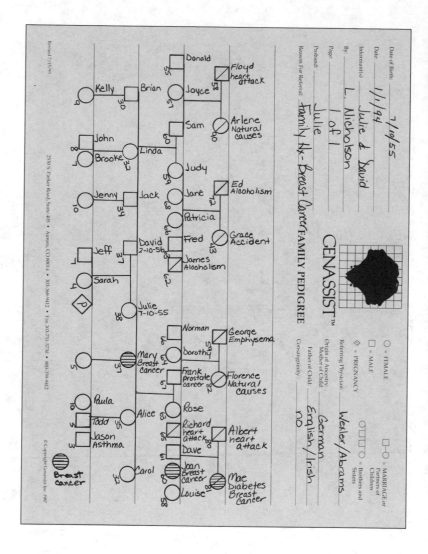

Figure 12 *Sample Pedigree. Note: hatched circles, showing recurrent cases of breast cancer.*

FETAL GROWTH

a. At what stage of pregnancy can you estimate how pregnant I am with ultrasound and if the baby is alive?

Many health care providers will want to perform a "size and dates" ultrasound usually between seven and nine weeks to measure the fetus, evaluate the viability of the pregnancy and calculate gestational dates with an error rate of (+/- 7 to 10 days). A "size and dates" ultrasound measures fetal position and viability, placenta location, and amniotic fluid volume. This procedure is by no means a national standard of care nor are doctors required to perform any ultrasound during a "normal" low risk pregnancy. Since many health care professionals will not schedule your first OB appointment until 10-11 weeks gestation, most "normal" pregnancies will not have a "size and dates" ultrasound.

Although most women are relatively sure as to their actual date of conception for a pregnancy, the health care professional always estimates dates from the first day of the last menstrual period unless the woman had a planned insemination, donor insemination, GIFT, ZIFT, or In-Vitro. A "size and dates" ultrasound can help the health care professional and the patient get accurate measurements of how the pregancy and the fetus are progressing during the pregnancy.

b. What is a Level II ultrasound of the fetus and when can it be done?

A Level II ultrasound, sometimes called a Level III ultrasound or a targeted ultrasound is a very careful ultrasound performed to evaluate the fetus and the progress of the pregnancy. A Level II ultrasound means that an M.D. either performs the study or the study is performed by an ultrasonographer and is read by an M.D. The Level II ultrasound usually takes 30-45 minutes depending upon how cooperative the fetus is. The Level II ultrasound is not performed until at least 15 weeks gestation, since the fetus' development has not progressed enough to accurately study with ultrasound. A Level II ultrasound can be done serially during the pregnancy if the health care professional wants to monitor a problem, or singly at any time during the pregnancy at or after 15 weeks gestation.

A Level II ultrasound is a critical survey of the fetal anatomy and includes:

1. Fetal head and its contents.
2. Fetal spine.
3. Kidneys.
4. Bladder.
5. Stomach.
6. Diaphragm.
7. Aortic arch.
8. 4 chamber view of the heart.
9. Right/left tibia and fibula.
10. Right/left femurs.
11. Right/left radius and ulna.
12. Placenta (location and integrity).
13. Umbilical cord insertion.
14. Number of vessels in the cord.
15. Volume of amniotic fluid.
16. Posterior fossa (where the spine and brain come together).
17. Internal cervical os (opening of the uterus).
18. A general survey of the fetus to note any irregularities.
19. Number and position of fetus.

c. How many weeks gestation before the heart is fully developed?

Although the heart is fully developed by 6 weeks after conception, its small size makes studying its compact chambers and valves very difficult. A comprehensive ultrasound study of the fetal heart can be performed between 20-24 weeks gestation (18-22 weeks following conception) and the study usually takes about one hour. This procedure is called Fetal Echocardiogram and evaluates:

1. The cardiac chambers.
2. Valves.
3. Valvular position.
4. Intraventricular septum.
5. Interatrial septum.
6. Foramenal flap insertion.
7. Position and size of great vessels (Aorta, pulmonary arteries).

8. Aortic arch.
9. Pericardiac space.
10. Contractibility of the muscle of the heart.

Indications for Fetal Echocardiogram: A family history in a first and/or second generation relative with congenital heart disease, renal or pulmonary anomalies, drug exposure (e.g. lithium, pergonal, dilantin, birth control pills), any anomalies of the fetal kidneys, idiopathic polyhydramnios (too much amniotic fluid) and diabetes mellitus. A Fetal Echocardiogram should be performed or read by an M.D.

d. How do I figure out how pregnant I am?

This question refers to the discrepancy between how far along the mother believes the pregnancy should be and the actual dates that are calculated by the ultrasound. If this discrepancy is greater than (+/- 7 to 10 days), or if part of the fetal anatomy measures out of proportion with the other fetal structure (e.g. a fetus that has a 16.1 weeks gestation head circumference and 16.5 weeks gestation stomach but a 12.1 weeks gestation femur length) this may mean that there is something wrong with the baby. Although there may not be anything wrong with the fetus, the health care professional will probably suggest serial ultrasound studies to monitor this discrepancy and see whether the dates get closer, stay the same or move farther apart as the pregnancy progresses. These studies are usually done at 4-6 week intervals. Remember, ultrasound requires a compilation of fetal measurements to give an estimated gestational age.

FETAL TISSUE

a. If I have a miscarriage or a stillborn infant can it be tested to see if there were abnormalities and whether I am at an increased risk in future pregnancies?

The stage of pregnancy when miscarriage occurs and the circumstances surrounding the miscarriage usually determines whether studies are performed. Since most pregnancies that will miscarry, miscarry in the first 11 weeks, it follows that many or most of the miscarriages occur before women know they are pregnant. After 11 weeks gestation the chance of evaluating a fetus after a miscarriage is greater. The further along the fetus is, the greater the chance that an examination and autopsy of the fetus may help rule out or identify abnormalities with the fetus or pregnancy. A genetics lab rarely ever gets fetal tissue from a miscarriage until after a pathologist at a hospital examined the fetus or baby. If the parents and the health care professional elect to, they can have chromosomal studies performed on the fetal tissue to identify or rule out possible chromosomal abnormalities. Sometimes, these studies help to support or rule out autopsy findings. These studies should only be requested if the results will be of benefit to the mother and/or her partner to help deal with their loss and help them prepare for the next pregnancy.

Later pregnancy losses and stillborns are more likely to be evaluated in order to identify the cause for the fetal death. In the state of Colorado, babies that miscarry after 20 weeks gestation or are stillborn must be examined by a medical examiner, pathologist or other physician to determine the cause of death. A death certificate must be filled out.

In order to properly evaluate whether a couple is at an increased risk for subsequent miscarriages or stillbirth a physical examination of the fetus as well as chromosomal evaluation of the fetus is recommended. The conditions in the pregnancy leading up to the loss must be reviewed. Just because a fetus miscarries or is stillborn does not necessarily mean that you are at a greater risk for recurrence in subsequent pregnancies. Your health care professional might suggest that you meet with a genetic or high risk obstetrical specialist to get a better idea as to recurrence risk.

b. Is it normal to have chromosome studies performed on a baby that miscarries? What steps do I need to take to make sure chromosome studies are performed?

NO, it is not routine to perform studies on a miscarriage. If a woman miscarries in a health care professional's office or in a hospital and products of conception can be collected by sterile methods the fetus will often be analyzed by a pathologist.

Usually, there are extenuating circumstances of the pregnancy or the family history of the patient that prompts further studies of the fetus. Special studies are only performed on the fetus if the patient and the referring doctor request them. A couple does not have to agree to have chromosomal studies performed on the fetus. In order to evaluate chromosomes of the fetus, tissue (membranes, skin, blood) of the fetus must be maintained in sterile saline. The lab only requires a little blood or skin of the fetus, otherwise the fetus remains intact.

Tissue Collection for Special Studies: Fetus or embryos, products of conception and amniotic membrane:

1. Collect tissue in a sterile container. If possible, transfer to a sterile container if not obtained aseptically. Sterile saline should be added to prevent drying.
2. If suction curretage is to be performed, attempt to obtain tissue with sterile ring or polyp forceps prior to the tissue passing through the suction tubing. The mixing of maternal blood with the tissue increases the risk of maternal contamination of the specimen.
3. **It is important not to add any substances which can injure live tissue (e.g. alcohol, formaldehyde).**
4. If available, the tissue can be examined by the pathologist and the fetus and/or embryo or chorionic villi can be separated from other tissue and transferred to a sterile container with saline or directly to culture media.
5. For large fetuses (greater than 20 weeks) a small amount of skin (minimally lacerated if possible) or kidneys or gonads should be obtained under sterile conditions and transfered to media with antibiotics and placed into a refrigerator until it can be picked up.

c. **If tissue is placed in formaldehyde and I change my mind about testing can the fetus still be tested?**

Tissue or products of conception in sterile saline in a refrigerator can last up to two weeks before it has to be prepared to be analyzed chromosomally. Once tissue is placed in formaldehyde a genetic lab has less than 12 hours to try to get any genetic study from the tissue. A full chromosomal karyotype usually can not be performed if formaldehyde has been added to the tissue, since it instantly kills live tissue.

For up to 12 hours following the addition of formaldehyde, it may be possible to perform a new test called Fluorescent In-Situ Hybridization (FISH) that can be used to identify or rule out abnormalities of chromosomes 13, 18, 21, X or Y. These are the more common abnormalities found in stillborn infants. After 12 hours, no genetic studies can be performed on the tissue within the limits of current technology.

d. What is fetal tissue research?

Fetal tissue research is the use of part or all of a fetus (i.e. ovaries, brain cells etc) for continued use in genetic research. For example, fetal cells from fetuses that have miscarried have been injected into the brains of Alzheimers' patients with some improvement in the patients. The ethical and moral ramifications of this research is endless. When you as parents or a couple agree to have genetic studies performed on your fetus or stillborn you should ask about and specify whether or not you agree to allow tissue research to be performed on the fetus. It is very much like a "Genetics Organ Donor" card. **If you object to additional use of the tissue beyond a chromosomal analysis, state that on the request for chromosome studies.** You have a right to allow all, part or none of your fetus to be analyzed. **If you want to have a funeral for your baby, state that at the time of the procedure, so that you will get the baby back.** This simple step should help prevent undo stress and heartache in an already unpleasant situation.

GENETIC CONSULTATION

a. What is a genetic consultation?

Usually genetic consultation can be divided into three parts:

1. The patient(s) and the genetic specialist or counsellor

     review family histories to determine whether there are any diseases which may recur in other relatives.

2. The genetics specialist or counsellor explains fully the risks for recurrence for diseases and conditions which have occurred in the family, and all tests and procedures that should be performed and why.

3. The patient gives written consent to have the procedures performed.

    The most important thing to remember during any genetic counseling session, is that this is a unique opportunity for you and your partner to ask and have questions answered which have concerned you about a previous pregnancy, this pregnancy or a future pregnancy.

GENETIC CONSULTATION LETTER EXAMPLE

2530 S. Parker Road
Suite #405
Aurora, CO 80014

Dear Dr. Smith,

I would like to thank you for the referral of your patient, Jane Doe seen on August 1, 1994 for prenatal genetic consultation. Attached you will find a copy of the family pedigree. We have highlighted the specific genetic issues that were identified in the family history. These are summarized below. Other family history issues which were identified are described in the pedigree.

ISSUE	ASSOCIATED RISK
Maternal age (33 years)	0.12%-0.20% for fetal chromosomal abnormality
Decreased AFP (0.44 MoM)	Increased risk (1:114) for trisomy 21 (Down syndrome)
Down syndrome - Maternal brother	Risk may be increased to 1% above age related risk
Cleft palate - paternal cousin	0.30% above the 3%-5% risk for a birth defect

Recommendations: The patient should be offered genetic amniocentesis since she has a low AFP with a Down syndrome risk of (1:114) and a first degree relative with Down syndrome.

We hope you find the above information helpful. If you have any additional questions or concerns, please do not hesitate to contact us. **Paul Wexler, M.D.**

---

b. When can a genetic consultation be performed?

Anytime. It is appropriate to seek genetic counseling as part of preconceptional planning if you have a known medical and/or genetic illness in the family, you are aware of some difficulties (e.g. recurrent miscarriage) which you have experienced in attempting to become pregnant or either you or your partner, are adopted or have an unknown family history. It is absolutely essential to have genetic counseling before any invasive procedures performed in pregnancy (i.e. CVS, amniocentesis). A consult is also helpful in the event that you are told that your fetus might be in danger of having an illness or problem. The consultation should help you to understand what diagnostic procedures you might chose in order to maximize the potential for the healthiest outcome for your pregnancy. After delivery, a genetic consultation can also be sought in the event that your child is thought to be developmentally delayed or to have a medical illness not diagnosed prenatally or specific congenital anomalies.

c. What is a genetic pedigree?

A genetic pedigree is a medical family tree which illustrates specific diseases or abnormalities that have affected various members of the family (See Genetic Pedigree Figure #12).

1. How is the genetic pedigree used medically?

It allows the counsellor to track the mode of inheritance of specific disorders in the family so that risks of recurrence in other family members can be calculated. It helps identify whether specific tests may help determine whether other family members do in fact have similar conditions or are likely to develop the problem. It helps to identify individuals in the family who should be studied if a condition in an affected individual is to be diagnosed.

d. Who can perform the genetic consultation?

Physicians, genetic counsellors, nurses, individuals with PhD's in genetics and other health care personnel specifically trained in analyzing a family history and researching genetic risks and making recommendations about specific testing or management of genetic problems.

INFECTIONS IN PREGNANCY

a. If I am diagnosed with an infection during my pregnancy, what type of prenatal diagnostic options do I have?

Having a cold or some other infection in pregnancy is very common. Although, it was believed that the placenta filtered bacteria and viruses from the baby's circulation, it is now known that the placenta offers little, if any, protection to the fetus.

Infections are most dangerous if they occur prior to the completion of the organ development of the fetus (approximately 9 weeks following conception). Fortunately, most infections do not cause malformations or miscarriage or infection in the fetus. Most bacterial infections will be handled by the woman's own immune system or antibiotics which are safe in pregnancy.

Viral infections such as german measles (rubella) can infect the placenta and fetus. Vaccination or natural infection with many viruses can offer significant and often lifelong protection against many of these agents. Specific antiviral therapy for example: Zovirax against herpes or varicella immune globulin (VZIG) against chicken pox may prevent or minimize the extent of the disease in the mother but the protection of the fetus is uncertain. Avoidance of individuals with known or undiagnosed infectious disease is recommended.

If an infection develops or a significant exposure to a known infectious agent occurs, you should contact your health care provider. Blood studies for prior infection (IGG- immunoglobulin G) and more recent infection (IGM - immuno-globulin

M) can help establish a diagnosis of the agent and a risk assessment can be made. This information might help the family and the health care provider to introduce monitoring of the fetal development and/or testing to help assure that significant harm to the fetus did not occur.

INFERTILITY: GIFT, ZIFT AND IN-VITRO

a. If I have infertility problems will my risk for abnormalities be increased?

Generally, the risks for abnormalities is not increased in couples that have problems conceiving. There are probably some couples in whom the failure to become pregnant is due to abnormal sperm and/or eggs which are less likely to fertilize or result in an abnormal conception which fails to implant. These couples will still fail to establish an identified pregnancy and will be considered to be infertile.

b. Are my risks for having an abnormal baby increased if I must use Assisted Reproductive Technology (e.g. GIFT, ZIFT, In-Vitro, donor egg, donor sperm, artificial insemination) to become pregnant?

Remarkably, most studies have suggested no increased risk for abnormal babies when these high tech procedures are used. A few studies have suggested a slightly increased risk (approximately 1%) for an abnormal child when any or all of these approaches are used. Because of this, some fertility programs recommend that women who have conceived with these approaches consider prenatal diagnosis.

c. If I use a donor egg, which age should I be concerned with, my age or that of the donor?

The use of a donor egg raises the same consideration for prenatal diagnosis as with any Assisted Reproductive Technique. However, the age of the woman donating the egg is probably the age which should be considered when calculating age related risk. The risks associated with Assisted Reproductive Techniques justifies offering prenatal diagnosis.

INSURANCE

a. What are insurance companies usual indications for prenatal diagnosis?

The American College of OB/GYN (ACOG) published prenatal guidelines in 1983 and revised them in 1986 to help establish indications for prenatal diagnosis. Prenatal diagnosis begins with a review of the woman's obstetrical and gynecological history as well as a complete review of all past medical history of both mother's and father's families. The purpose of reviewing family history is to attempt to identify conditions or symptoms or specific diseases/disorders for which a child and/or the pregnancy may be at risk.

Screening in pregnancy by counselling, CVS, amniocentesis or ultrasound is strongly recommended if any of the following apply to you:

1. You are a pregant woman over 35 years of age or younger than 20 years of age.
2. You or your partner have a history of having a previous child with an abnormality.
3. You are a woman with a history of two or more spontaneous miscarriages.
4. You are a woman with a history of a diagnosable abnormality in either your family or that of your partner, in a grandparent, parent, brother, sister, niece or nephew, aunt or uncle or first or second cousin.

5. You or your partner is a carrier or is affected by a sex-linked disorder (e.g. Duchenne Muscular Dystrophy, Hemophilia).
6. You or your partner are carriers of an inborn error of metabolism (e.g. Tay Sachs, Phenylketonuria (PKU).
7. You or your partner has a serious medical disease (e.g. Epilepsy, Diabetes)
8. You are man over 45 years of age and your partner is pregnant.
9. You have had an abnormal result on a prenatal test (e.g. AFP, AFP3, Ultrasound).
10. You or your partner have a known chromosomal abnormality.

b. Do all insurance companies follow these indications? If not, why?

No. Most insurance companies accept most of the above guidelines, however, companies that are self insured have the right to make their own list and exclude any or all of the above list as long as each employee is notified at the time he/she seeks employment and health insurance. The above list is a suggested guideline but no federal or state laws have mandated this list as the only acceptable standard of care. The most common reason for not following these guidleines is the "pre-existing" clause in many insurance contracts.

The pre-existing clause lasts between six months and two years after the subscriber (employee) enrolls in an insurance plan. During this time if the employee has any injury, pregnancy or illness that requires diagnosis and medical treatment it could be considered "pre-existing". Many employers join HMO's (health maintenance organizations) or PPO's (preferred provider organizations) and follow the HMO's or PPO's guidelines for prenatal diagnosis. It is always best for the employee to talk with their subscriber relations person (the person who manages the employee's health insurance for the company) prior to seeking treatment, to see if the services will be covered or whether the services will be considered pre-existing and not covered. Most insurance companies have a disclaimer that is read to a physician or hospital at the time of service that states that they can not guarantee payment or eligibility of the claim until the time that the claim is received. By that time is can be too late for the employee. The insurance companies will provide the subscriber (employee) with deductible, coinsurance, pre-existing, eligibility and plan provisions but more often than not, they will not provide this information to the doctor or hospital performing your services.

IN-UTERO SURGERY

a. What is in-utero surgery?

In-utero surgery is a technique that allows physicians to surgically repair or correct certain physical defects of the fetus, while it is still in the uterus of the pregnant mother. Although, most physical abnormalities will be surgically repaired or corrected after delivery, there are a few conditions that give the fetus little to no chance of survival without in-utero surgery.

In a recent article in Denver, there was a couple that had a fetus with a diaphragmatic hernia in which the diaphragm had a hole in it and allowed the intestines to grow into the chest cavity. This defect prevented the normal growth of the fetal lungs. These babies appear normal at birth but die soon afterwards due to immature lungs. The diaphragmatic hernia was detected prenatally by ultrasound. The patient and her partner were offered the option of trying in-utero surgery to correct the defect, or face the reality of a very low survival rate if the surgery was deferred until the newborn period.

The couple elected to proceed with the surgery. This story has a tragic ending. Although the surgery itself did correct the abnormality, the baby died 15 days after delivery due to an infection unrelated to the surgery. This case has raised moral and ethical discussions as well as insurance issues since the care cost over $2,000,000. Medical societies and the insurance companies are reviewing what financial cost is too much to save a child. Most parents would say that they would give up almost anything to save their child. With managed health care and the threat of national health care reform, parents are going to be forced to make tougher and tougher financial decisions that will affect the outcome of their pregnancy.

Experimental prenatal surgery centers are reviewing the cost, benefits and outcome from these surgeries. Many surgical teams have abandoned these techniques due to the high costs and the low survival rates of the babies. Even if the surgery is successful, many of these children can have permanent injury following the procedures. This is technology that will quickly be forgotten if society decides the outcome is not worth the cost. Most people feel that unless someone else is paying for these high tech approaches to health care, it is a luxury most of us can not afford.

LABORATORY

a. How long should test results take?

When prenatal diagnosis started in 1972, the issue of turnaround time for test results was not very important. Many programs took 8-12 weeks for amniocentesis results and a few programs even waited for the delivery of the baby before test results were given. Since then public and health care provider pressure and new laboratory techniques, has led to more rapid results. The following describes the approximate time from the specimen acquisition to the final report:

1. **AFP** - Maternal serum AFP or amniotic fluid AFP results usually take 24 hours to one week.
2. **AFP3** - The triple screen (AFP, beta HCG and estriol) results may be ready as soon as 48-72 hours; a few programs are batching the tests and only call results out every 10-14 days.
3. **Amniocentesis** - Amniotic fluid chromosome results can be reported as soon as six days. Most are reported between eight and ten days following the procedure. Occassionally, it can take up to 14 or 15 days to get a result. This does not mean that there is anything wrong with your baby. Most labs will check all specimens on day six or seven following the procedure to

determine if an early result can be obtained. (Remember: Normal cells grow at different rates).

4. **Blood Chromosomes** - Adult, child, newborn and umbilical cord blood chromosome studies are usually reported in 5-7 days, but can take as long as 10-14 days depending on growth.

5. **Chorionic Villus Sampling (CVS)** - Although all CVS specimens are studied the day of or the day following the procedure, most laboratories have determined that the most reliable results are obtained when the first day examination is combined with the results obtained from the culture. These results are usually available in 5-10 days following the procedure.

6. **DNA/Special Tests** - Each of these test results will vary by the test requested and the lab performing the test. Check with your heath care provider **before** the specimen is sent as to which lab was selected to do the work, the turnaround time for results and the cost of the test.

b. What are the most common genetic abnormalities seen in the lab?

Contrary to popular belief, Down syndrome is not the most common abnormality seen in a genetics lab. The most common genetic abnormalities are sex chromosomal abnormalities in which there are too many sex chromosomes (e.g 47,XXY; 47,XXX or 47,XYY) or too few chromosomes (e.g. Turner syndrome 45,XO). Aneuploidies which describes abnormal numbers of chromosomes other than sex chromosomes (e.g. Down syndrome 47,XX,+21 or 47,XY,+21) are seen next most common Translocations, where parts of certain chromosomes break off and reattach with other chromosomes (e.g. 46,XY t(13;14) or 46,XY t(9;22)). The t(13;14) means that all or part of the #13 chromosome has broken off and exchanged material with all or part of the #14 chromosome. In the second example, chromosome #9 and #22 have exchanged material.

c. How many cells do you count for a normal karyotype? An abnormal karyotype?

A minimum of 10-15 cells are counted for a normal karyotype. At least two of the three cultures of the specimen are reviewed. When a specimen is drawn it is usually separated into three or four vials or specimens denoted as Side A, Side B and Side C. For an abnormal karyotype in which all the cells studied have the same abnormality a minimum of 15 cells are read. As many as 100 cells may be reviewed to confirm the abnormality. All three sides (A side, B side and C side) are read to confirm the abnormality.

d. How do you decide when results are finished?

A case is considered to be finished when the laboratory supervisor and the medical director feel that the sample tested is accurately representative of the cells which are present in the CVS or amniotic fluid.

e. How do you know the cells that are sampled are from my baby?

When amniocentesis was first developed, cultures from the mother's blood were set up and studied parallel with the amniotic fluid culture. Both the mother's cells and the amniotic fluid cells had chromosomal studies performed to rule out possible maternal contamination. Studies were performed on umbilical cord blood at the birth of the baby to confirm that the cells tested were the cells of the baby. Most labs do not perform these parallel tests today since the certainty of the test results were established in the early years of the procedure.

f. When a laboratory says that they have ruled out greater than 99% of the known chromosomal abnormalities for a normal karyotype what does that mean?

It means that the lab has ruled out all chromosomal abnormalities involving extra or missing chromosomes or parts of chromosomes and no material has been exchanged between chromosomes. Among these are approximately 100 named chromosomal diseases and/or syndromes. Potentially, there are an unlimited number of things that can go wrong chromosomally and might not yet have been described. New syndromes and abnormalities of the chromosomes continue to be described.

LICENSURE

a. Are genetics companies federally licensed and regulated? What does that mean?

Most if not all of the laboratories across the country that handle human specimens are federally licensed and regulated to ensure quality and accuracy of testing. Once a lab becomes clinical and/or diagnostic the lab must apply for the following types of licenses:

1. **Certificate of Waiver:** A certificate or license that allows a doctor to perform a limited panel of tests that are considered waived of federal regulations.
2. **Certificate For Physician Performed Microscopy Procedures:** A certificate or license that allows a doctor to perform tests in his/her office.
3. **Certificate of Accreditation:** A certificate or license that allows a doctor or laboratory to perform laboratory tests. As part of this accreditation, labs are required or encouraged (rules vary by state) to permit unannounced site visits by state or federal inspectors, be part of a proficiency testing program for each of the tests performed in the lab (either monthly, quarterly, semiannually or annually) and participate in a quality control program for accredited labs.

In order for a laboratory to be considered to be federally licensed and regulated the lab must meet or exceed all federal and state quality assurance standards. Licenses are issued for two years but are not automatically renewed every two years. The license can be rescinded by the federal regulating body at any time if the laboratory falls below proficiency standards.

b. What is CLIA? When was it passed?

CLIA stands for the Clinical Laboratory Improvement Amendments Act which was passed by Congress on October 31, 1988, interpreted and implemented by the Health Care Financing Administration (HCFA) in February 1992, and signed into law by President George Bush in September 1992. CLIA is the law that led to the federal licensing and regulation of all laboratories including private doctors' offices that handle human specimens.

c. What is proficiency testing for a lab?

Under CLIA, all labs that perform a given test are periodically screened to make sure that the results of each lab are comparable to the majority of the other labs. In order to do this the following steps are taken:

1. Controls are sent out to all participating labs to be tested.
2. The samples must be tested and returned in a timely manner or will not be considered (a definite date of return is labelled on each specimen). Any specimen postmarked after the return date is disqualified.
3. The lab is rated on overall score and accuracy of the test results.
4. If the proficiency of any test falls below 75% then the lab can be placed on probation. If the lab fails to correct the cause of the problem it will remain on probation and/or risk having its license suspended or revoked. These tests are taken very seriously by the labs since it can mean the difference between keeping their doors open or closing.

MISCARRIAGE

a. What is the miscarriage risk for a normal pregnancy?

Even if a pregnant mother does not have any invasive procedures during the pregnancy, at least 15%-20% of pregnancies miscarry. Up to 60% of early miscarriages will demonstrate some abnormality of the chromosomes. As pregnancy progresses the miscarriage rate falls. At 15-17 weeks, the time when amniocentesis is performed, at least 1%-2% of pregnancies will still be lost spontaneously.

b. What is the miscarriage risk following CVS, early amniocentesis and amniocentesis?

The miscarriage risk for CVS is approximately 1%-2% above the general population's risk for miscarriage. The miscarriage risk for both early amniocentesis and amniocentesis is approximately 1:200-1:500 (0.20%-0.50%) procedures performed with direct vision (use of ultrasound guidance) over the general population's miscarriage risk.

c. How many miscarriages should I have before I have genetic studies performed on myself and/or partner?

The literature is divided. Some programs believe that after three or more miscarriages (even if a normal birth occurred between losses), blood chromosome studies of both parents should be performed to rule out a possible chromosomal abnormality. Other programs believe that after only two miscarriages parents should consider having blood chromosomes performed. With a history of multiple pregnancy losses there is a 4%-7% incidence that either parent may have abnormal chromosomes which can be diagnosed by blood chromosome studies. Since patients and/or their partners who carry a chromosomal abnormality have an increased incidence of giving birth to a baby with a chromosomal abnormality (5%-10%) and/or of additional pregnancy losses, it is advisable to encourage these parents to consider prenatal diagnosis (CVS or amniocentesis) because of their increased incidence of carrying a child with a chromosomal abnormality to term.

Additional literature suggests that women with recurrent pregnancy losses also may have lupus anticoagulant and/or anticardiolipin antibodies in their blood. Data suggests that many of these patients with these abnormal antibodies can be treated successfully with medication to increase the likelihood of carrying a baby to term. Neither blood chromosomes nor studies for lupus anticoagulant and/or anticardiolipin are considered experimental.

d. Does having a history of miscarriage increase my risk of having a miscarriage following CVS, early amniocentesis or amniocentesis?

Although, there is no data proving an increased risk for

miscarriage for these patients following these procedures, it is reasonable to assume that the miscarriage risk is greater than for a woman who has never miscarried.

e. How long after the procedure of CVS, early amniocentesis and amniocentesis should miscarriage be attributed to the procedure?

Most patients who are going to miscarry following the procedure will do so in the first 14 days. Spotting or bleeding, cramping, loss of fluid or decreased fetal movement are all indications of a possible problem. Amniocentesis or CVS providers are supposed to document miscarriage within 30 days following the procedure. The reason for 30 days is that unless complications arise during the first 30 days following an invasive procedure, the miscarriage was probably NOT caused by the procedure. Oftentimes, CVS or amniocentesis is performed on pregnancies already at increased risk for miscarriage (e.g. multiple fetuses, little or no fluid, fetuses with abnormalities, patients with cramping and/or bleeding prior to the procedure). The 30 day rule is a common rule applied by most doctors to attribute complications and/or problems to any invasive procedure. After this time, other causes are sought to explain a negative outcome.

NEWBORN TESTING

a. What tests are routinely performed on newborn babies?

Most metabolic disorders are inherited in an autosomal recessive manner. Both parents would have to be gene carriers of the abnormal gene and both parents would have to pass the abnormal gene on to the baby for the baby to be affected.

Different states screen newborn babies differently. Your child will usually be screened in the newborn period for one or more of the following diseases:

1. **Biotinidase deficiency:** Biotin is a water soluble vitamin belonging to the Vitamin B complex group. Deficiency of the enzyme biotinidase is inherited in an autosomal recessive manner and may affect approximately 1:70,000 births. If untreated, the condition can result in hypotonia (weakness), seizures, breathing or balance problems and developmental delay. The disease can be very variable. If discovered early, children can be treated with biotin and diet modification will usually prevent the problems described from developing.

2. **Cystic Fibrosis (CF):** Cystic Fibrosis is the most common fatal autosomal recessive disease that affects the white population and may affect 1:1800 newborns. Although the clinical symptoms can be quite variable the most seriously affected will demonstrate obstruction of the lungs with subsequent infection, poor weight gain in childhood, chronic illness, digestive problems with possible obstruction of the bowel and sterility in males may occur. New work suggests that less common changes in an individual's DNA may result in milder problems which may not become evident until adulthood. New treatment including possible gene therapy should improve the survival rate of the most seriously affected individuals who had a less than 50% chance of surviving into their 40's.

3. **Galactosemia:** Galactosemia is inherited in an autosomal recessive manner. Several different inherited problems can result in galactosemia. Problems can vary from cataracts alone to failure to thrive, weight loss, vomiting, liver problems and mental retardation. The disease is quite rare affecting only 1 in 20,000-40,000 people. Dietary management is required.

4. **Homocystinuria:** Homocystinuria is inherited in an autosomal recessive manner with a frequency of approximately 1 in 335,000 births. Mild and more severe cases have been described resulting in tall stature, dislocation of the ocular lens, seizures, mental retardation, thinning of bones and blood clotting. Vitamin treatment (pyridoxine) will help some patients but not others. Dietary management is usually employed.

5. **Hypothyroidism/Hyperthyroidism:** This test is really designed to pick up hypothyroidism. Hypothyroidism is an underactive thyroid condition and hyperthyroidsim is an overactive thyroid. Undiagnosed underactive thyroid activity occurs in approximately 1 in 4000 births and can result in developmental delay and/or mental retardation which will not respond to thyroid treatment unless treatment is introduced shortly after birth. Even with treatment normalcy of the patient is not assured. Hyperthyroidism is associated with increased heart rate and can usually be treated with medication.

6. **Maple Syrup Urine Disease (MSUD):** Maple Syrup Urine Disease has an incidence of between 1:760 for certain inbred populations to approximately 1:300,000. Maple Syrup Urine Disease is inherited in an autosomal recessive manner. Dietary management including synthetic products and vitamin (thiamine) supplements can almost always avoid the seizures, coma, physical and mental retardation and possible death which may result with delayed diagnosis and treatment.

7. **Phenylketonuria (PKU):** Phenylketonuria is inherited in an autosomal recessive manner. The disease incidence varies in different parts of the world (1 or 2 in 190 million births) and the severity also varies. Symptoms may include simple elevation in blood levels of phenylalanine with no adverse affects to impaired growth, small head, mental retardation and malformations. Early recognition and treatment has allowed a substantial number of women to reach childbearing age and conceive. Careful dietary regulation can result in near normal or normal infants.

8. **Sickle Cell Anemia (SCA):** Sickle Cell Anemia is an autosomal recessive disease which originated in individuals of African descent. Because of the wide migration from Africa, Sickle Cell Anemia and some variants can be found throught the world with some areas of increased prevalence (e.g. the Mediterranean region, the Middle East, and India). The major problems associated with the disease are anemia and/or

clotting of vessels and an increased risk for infection. Aggressive treatment of severe anemia, in which large numbers of red blood cells become "sickle-shaped" causing pain and/or clotting and recognition and treatment of infection appear to be lowering the mortality from this disease.

You will probably not even be aware of these tests unless your baby tests positive for any of the above list. The list of tests may vary from hospital to hospital but you can call before you go into the hospital to get a list of the things that they screen for. Since we never heard from the hospital about these tests, we assume that Haylee tested negative for all of these. What alerted us to finding this list, was when a friend of our's, who recently delivered a child, was called at home by the hospital and told that her child had tested positive for Cystic Fibrosis. The hospital needed more blood from the baby so the lab could confirm or rule out the diagnosis of Cystic Fibrosis.

Needless to say, she and her partner were a little shocked to find out not only that their child had been tested and they were not aware of the testing but now their beautiful newborn might have Cystic Fibrosis. The second test was performed on her child and the second screen was negative for Cystic Fibrosis. This example should serve as reminder to expectant parents to ask what tests your baby will be screened for so that if a result comes back positive, you will have had time to prepare for it.

b. How reliable are these test results?

To date, of the thousands of pregnancies that deliver each year in Colorado, the laboratory at Genassist, Inc. has only been contacted by three patients whose children tested positive for one of the above tests. Obviously, other children have been tested elsewhere. If a child tests positive for any of the above tests, a more reliable and accurate second test will be run to confirm the diagnosis or rule out a false positive. Of the three patients who tested positive on the first test none have tested positive on the second test.

PATERNITY TESTING

a. What is paternity testing?

Paternity testing is used to confirm who is the biological father of a child. With the issue of legal heirs to estates, paternity suits, surrogacy and adoption cases, studies can be performed to establish either maternity or paternity (the biological mother or father of a child).

b. Can you perform paternity testing on amniotic fluid or CVS?

Yes. Paternity testing can be performed on amniotic fluid or CVS prenatally, although most labs performing these tests prefer to do the testing once the baby is born. There are two reasons for this:

1. The reliability of the test is more accurate on newborns than prenatally.
2. Most states will not legally force a suspected "father" of a child to have his blood drawn for paternity studies until the child has been born. Likewise, to do paternity testing prenatally a mother must either have amniocentesis or CVS to obtain fetal cells to be tested. Most mothers do not want to incur the expense (since the amniocentesis for paternity is not covered by insurance) nor the risk of miscarriage from the procedure.

c. How many family members do you need to perform paternity testing?

Paternity testing can not be performed without at least three people: the biological mother, the fetus or baby and the suspected biological father. Since paternity testing is a comparison study of the mother's and father's red and white blood cells in relationship to the cells of the fetus or baby, this causal relationship can not be established if only one parent is studied. These tests are very specialized and are performed only by a few laboratories since the test results are admissable in a court of law, and the lab must provide experts to explain the test results. The cost for paternity testing is at least $160-$200 per specimen multiplied by at least three people (the biological mother, the fetus or baby and the suspected biological father). There are usually additional charges for expert testimony in court.

PREIMPLANTATION GENETICS

a. What is preimplantation genetics? How reliable are the results?

This is a very new and exciting and somewhat controversial field of genetics. Unlike traditional prenatal diagnosis by CVS, early amniocentesis or amniocentesis to get a chromosomal karyotype of the fetus, some couples are choosing to have chromosome analysis performed at the time of the ZIFT or In-Vitro procedure. Since the egg and sperm are already being manipulated during these procedures, the time of conception is precise, and the cells are constantly monitored for cellular divisions. As early as the 3rd cell divison called the eight cell stage, a single cell can be removed, usually without jeopardizing the integrity of the fertilized egg (embryo). This single cell can be set up like CVS or amniocentesis cells in media and allowed to grow and divide. In theory, this single cell should give an expectant couple an accurate karyotype of the chromosomes of the fetus before the fertilized egg or eggs are replaced in the mother.

There are a number of reasons why women are not rushing out and having preimplantation genetics performed:

1. Depending upon where in the country a couple has ZIFT or In-Vitro performed, the cost for an infertility treatment cycle is $3500-$10,000. For example, if a woman has 12 eggs surgically removed and fertilized to be used in future attempts at getting pregnant, each fertilized egg (embryo) would have to be separately analyzed before replacement. Most genetics labs are currently charging $350-$1000 per specimen. The cost for such studies becomes very great.

2. Only those embryos that are chromosomally normal would be reimplanted. Abnormal embryos would be

discarded. However, even at the eight cell stage of division, the chromosomal results are only 75% accurate as to the final genetic chromosomal karyotype of the fetus. The reason for this is because only a single cell is being tested, and an abnormal cell line that is present in one or all of the seven other cells might not be detected. Additionally, an abnormality in one or more cells could develop after replacement.

3. Even if a normal karyotype is given at the time of the ZIFT or In-Vitro procedure, the couple usually will be offered CVS, early amniocentesis or amniocentesis to confirm the results. Preimplantation genetics can not rule out possible physical abnormalities that might occur, so the couple should be offered a maternal serum AFP between 14 and 22 weeks gestation as well as a Level II ultrasound after 15 weeks gestation.

At the time of this publication there were two new techniques that were being used and showing great promise for the future applications of preimplantation genetics. One research group published a paper showing that they had been able to detect abnormal cell lines in the dividing fertilized embryos, and were able to repair the embryos by removing the abnormal cells and allowing only the normal ones to continue to divide. These corrected "normal" embryos were then reimplanted. This study was done on animals not on humans, but may pave the way for earlier and more accurate genetic preimplantation diagnosis.

Several research groups have announced that they are capable of doing carrier testing on the embryo prior to implanting it. These groups were able to detect the first embryo that was affected with Tay Sachs disease. Only the embryos that tested negative for Tay Sachs were replaced. The abnormal embryos that tested positive for the Tay Sachs gene were discarded. Recently, the list of disorders which might be diagnosed in this way has been expanded.

This research is partially financed by federal grants from the National Institute of Health (NIH). Even with federal grants this procedure costs between $6500-$7500 per cycle (the cost is shared between the federal grant fiscal limitations and the patient) and is dependent upon whether the disease or trait that affects the family is detectable. At present the patient must travel to the state that the preimplantation genetics lab is in, for each cycle of treatment. The couple usually must stay at least 5-7 days. There are no guarantees that you will get pregnant from this procedure and the results are still considered experimental pending federal review.

PRENATAL TESTING

a. What is the general population's risk of having a child with a birth defect?

3% to 5%. Only 1%-2% of these birth defects are considered major and will seriously affect the life and/or health of the child.

b. What is maternal/fetal blood screening?

Maternal/Fetal blood screening is the ability to take blood from a pregnant mother and separate the cells of the fetus from the mother's cells so that the fetal cells can be analyzed for chromosomal defects. To date, although a tremendous amount of money has been spent towards perfecting this technology **no laboratory has been able to reliably and repeatedly separate maternal cells from the fetal cells.** If this technique is ever perfected it will provide a safer option than CVS or amniocentesis since the mother will only have to have blood drawn from her arm instead of having an invasive procedure performed. Given this "safer" and less invasive option, most health care professionals believe that most or all pregnancies would be screened genetically in the future.

c. What is Fluorescent In-Situ Hybridization (F.I.S.H.)?

F.I.S.H. is a relatively new technology that can assist laboratories in identifying and/or confirming chromosomal abnormalities (i.e. too many chromosomes, too few chromosomes or parts of chromosomes being lost, being duplicated or exchanging with other chromosomes). F.I.S.H. is a fancy name for "painting" all or parts of chromosomes (with a fluorescent dye).

F.I.S.H. is valuable in confirming or helping to further evaluate a possible karyotype abnormality. Each F.I.S.H probe (fluorescent marker) is specific to an entire chromosome or a piece of chromosome and will show up only on the chromosomes or parts of the specific chromosome for which the probe was designed.

F.I.S.H. technology is also helpful in providing at least a limited genetic study (usually chromosome 13, 18, 21, X and Y) for tissue that has been placed in formalydehyde. Before F.I.S.H., if a specimen was placed in formaldehyde no genetic studies could be performed. The one limitation at present is that the probes can only paint or fluoresce tissue that has been placed in formaldehyde up to 12 hours. After that time the probes will not attach to the chromosomes, and the genetic study is useless. The reason why most labs are only using F.I.S.H. technology sparingly is because each chromosomal probe costs between $100 and $150. For a study to be performed with F.I.S.H. you would need 22 probes for chromosomes 1-22 and an X and a Y probe. The total cost of the procedure would be approximately $2500 for the probes alone. In Colorado, a genetic consultation and amniocentesis with a Level II ultrasound cost approximately $1160. Additionally, even when different colors for each of the chromosomes are available, interpretation of overlapping chromosomes will make interpretation difficult and probably more costly.

d. Can you detect mental retardation, cerebral palsy or multiple sclerosis prenatally?

Mental retardation might be detected prenatally if associated with a chromosomal syndrome (i.e. Down syndrome). The severity of the mental retardation can not be estimated until the child is old enough to be evaluated. Cerebral palsy can be caused by a variety of factors including birth trauma and can not be detected prenatally. Multiple sclerosis is a late onset disease in which symptoms usually do not appear until teens or twenties and therefore can not be diagnosed prenatally.

RECURRENCE RISK

a. If I had an abnormal baby previously, what is my recurrence risk?

Many diseases are not inherited and the risk for recurrence in a subsequent pregnancy is no higher than in normal subsequent pregnancies. However, if there is an inherited component to the disease the risk of recurrence is usually broken into four categories:

Autosomal dominant, autosomal recessive, X-linked and multifactorial.

1. **Autosomal dominant** - If a disease manifests itself when only one abnormal gene is inherited from one parent it is called autosomal dominant. This risk may approach 50% in some families.

2. **Autosomal recessive** - This defines a disease which manifests itself only if the same abnormal gene is inherited from both parents. This risk may approach 25% in some families.

3. **X-linked recessive inheritance** - Since a male has only one X chromosome and one Y chromosome, an abnormal gene on the X chromosome may result in a disease. Since a female has two X chromosomes, the effect of the abnormal X may be offset by the normal gene on the other X chromosome. Rarely, a single abnormal gene on one X chromosome in a female will result in a disease. When this occurs, the disease is usually milder than it is in the male. The disease is usually passed from a carrier female to her children. 50% of male children would be affected, 50% of females would be carriers.

4. **Multifactorial inheritance** - This mode of inheritance occurs when there is an interaction between a genetic predisposition and environmental factors which result in a certain disease. Certain families have a greater probability that environmental factors will result in a disease. The risk for recurrence is 2%-5%.

These are the four major categories that are used to give a risk for recurrence for genetic diseases. Depending upon the disease or trait, there are a variety of combinations of any or all of the above categories to help establish a risk. The reason that genetic consultation is suggested to help establish recurrence risk, is that the recurrence risk will vary family by family. Each recurrence risk will be unique to each family that is analyzed. These risks provide a statistical analysis of possible risks for recurrence for a particular disorder in a family. This is not a guarantee that a disorder will or will not recur.

RH FACTOR

a. What is Rh sensitization?

Rh sensitization occurs when a mother with Rh negative blood type is exposed to Rh positive blood cells from the fetus and the mother becomes "sensitized". This means that a woman develops antibodies (protein that can cross the placenta and cause anemia in the fetus) as a response to the Rh positive red blood from the fetus in her circulation. When the mother has an Rh negative blood type and the child has an Rh positive blood type, the sensitization occurs due to incompatible blood types between the mother and child. When a mother becomes sensitized all subsequent pregnancies are at a greater risk for spontaneous abortion, neonatal death and complications in the fetus due to anemia. Women that have Rh negative blood and a partner with Rh positive blood are given an injection of Rh-immune globulin (Rhogam) after any invasive procedure during pregnancy to avoid sensitization since the fetal blood type will not be known until delivery. At delivery, if the baby is Rh positive the mother receives another injection of Rhogam.

b. What is Rhogam?

Rhogam is a drug called Rh-immune globulin that can be administered to pregnant women with an Rh negative blood type to prevent them from being sensitized to an Rh positive blood type fetus. In order to avoid sensitization, Rhogam which is usually administered by injection, is given within 72 hours **after** an invasive procedure. Rhogam shots are usually repeated at 28 weeks gestation and post delivery.

SEXING YOUR BABY

a. Can a baby's sex be determined in pregnancy by ultrasound? What is the reliability?

Yes. Most programs will not perform ultrasound studies simply to determine the sex of your baby, even if you offer to pay for the entire study yourself. Having an ultrasound study to determine the sex of a fetus is not considered medically necessary, and will most likely not be covered by your insurance. Although fetal sex can usually be determined correctly using ultrasound (up to 96% accuracy) there is always the possibility of error. Since ultrasound is a computer enhanced picture based upon sound waves that are bounced off your baby, the picture you see of the baby is not an x-ray, but rather a computer's interpretation of the sound that it receives. Determining the sex of your baby depends upon the position of the fetus, the quality of the ultrasound equipment and the skill of the health care provider performing the study.

b. How reliable is determination of my baby's sex by chromosome studies?

Virtually 100%. A fetus is either a boy (46,XY), a girl (46,XX), or the sex chromosomes are abnormal. Sex determination is one of the first things that a genetics lab looks for to rule out sex chromosomal abnormalities. Because CVS samples the placenta and not fetal cells directly, there is a small chance for error (less than 1%-2%). Placental chromosomes may not be identical with fetal chromosomes.

SEX SELECTION - PRECONCEPTIONAL

a. What is preconceptional sex selection?

Preconceptional sex selection refers to the technique of using laboratory manipulation of husband's or partner's sperm (both male determining (Y) and female determining (X) exist in a sperm specimen) to attempt to conceive a child of a desired sex

(sex selection). Great interest exists regarding the possibility of increasing the chances for having a child of a particular sex. Several methods have been explored and many researchers are continuing to investigate the safety and likelihood of success for current methods as well as explore easier, less costly and more certain methods for guaranteeing the sex of a particular pregnancy.

All of the preconceptional sex selection methods are investigational. Neither the success nor safety can be guaranteed. No work done to date has indentified any significant risk for these methods to either the mother or the child conceived as a result of these manipulations. Spinning specimens at high speed, special filters and passing sperm through special solutions have all been described as methods to enhance the ratio of one particular sex over the other. These methods have been used successfully by researchers with a 75%-80% likelihood that the sex selected will be the one that is conceived. However, other laboratories have abandoned these techniques as their statistics began to approach those of spontaneous pregnancies.

Many programs use these above laboratory manipulations in conjuction with ultrasound studies to evaluate the size of the ovarian follicles, artificial insemination, and may require the use of a fertility drug such as Clomid (Serophene) and HCG (human chorionic gonadotropin) to be able to better predict the ovulation and enhance the pregnancy rate. Below is an **example of a consent form for Sperm Separation For Sex Selection:**

I have agreed to the laboratory manipulations of my husband's/partner's semen to attempt to conceive a child of a desired sex (sex selection). I understand that even if I have been able to conceive in the past, my chances are greatly reduced using sex selection due to the separation of the semen specimen into males and females and the corresponding ratio and motility of each.

Although there are no studies to indicate that these methods for sperm separation are dangerous, I realize that these methods are new and experimental, and no guarantees have been made regarding a successful outcome. I have only a 17% chance each cycle to conceive (these statistics may vary from program to program).

I realize that 3%-5% of all infants born have birth defects and that my child conceived with or without sperm separation might have a birth defect.

I also realize that manipulation of sperm and/or eggs may result in an increased incidence of miscarriage or abnormal children, although the absolute risks for these problems or whether these manipulations may increase my risk for having an abnormal child are unknown.

I realize that CVS or amniocentesis is advisable, which may diagnose birth defects due to a chromosomal defect and can also diagnose the sex of the child.

I understand that sex selection is an elective procedure and insurance will not cover the procedure.

---

b. Why do laboratories perform sex selection?

Preconceptional sex selection was created to help those parents that either are affected or are known carriers of an abnormal gene which can cause an inborn error of metabolism in a male child or a X-linked recessive disorder which affects males (e.g. Duchenne Muscular Dystrophy, Hemophilia). Since the disease discriminates on the basis of sex in which up to 50% of males might be affected and 50% of females would only be carriers of the disease, many couples would like to limit their chances of having an affected child by attempting sex selection with a 75%-80% success rate. Until the creation of preconceptional sex selection, parents who had a genetic predisposition that would affect one sex but not the other had only a few options:

1. Never attempt to have a child themselves.
2. Ignore the problem, try to conceive, and hope that the child is not the sex that is affected by this disease knowing that up to 50% of that sex will be affected.
3. Seek a surrogate mother, or donor egg, or donor sperm.
4. Have prenatal diagnosis using CVS or amniocentesis to determine the sex of the child.

That was the reason that the technology was created. However, like most good ideas that is not how the technology has been used. The majority of the preconceptional sex selection cases are for parents that simply want a little boy or a little girl. Labs across the country have made a conscious decision about whether to offer preconceptional sex selection to couples that do not have a medical indication.

TEST RESULTS - ABNORMALS

a. If I am told that my baby has an abnormality, what do I do with the information?

One of the most painful and difficult times for an expectant parent(s) is when the joy of being future parents is burst by the prospect of an abnormality. There is never a good time to receive bad news. However, when an abnormality is found prenatally tough decisions have to be made. As an expectant parent you must ask your health care professional the difficult questions regarding the prognosis for your child. We have provided a list of suggestions for questions that can be asked to help you compile enough information so that you and your partner can make educated and well informed decisions:

1. Never allow a health care professional or lab to give you an abnormal result and not be able to meet with you and discuss the abnormality. If this happens, asked to be referred to someone who can answer your questions or seek a second opinion.
2. If the problem is a structural abnormality find out which organ(s) of the fetus are affected (i.e. intestines, brain, spine) and to what extent any or all of the structures are affected.

   a. Ask what the prognosis is for the survival of the fetus?
   b. Can the problem be corrected or repaired with surgery? If so, what if any are the additional risks to the baby?
   c. What is the probability that mental retardation or brain impairment is present or is likely to be present following the attempts to correct the problem?
   d. Will the baby be paralyzed?
   e. Are chromosomal abnormalities associated with these structural problems?
   f. Is it safer for the baby to be delivered vaginally or by C-section?
   g. Will I have to deliver at a certain hospital?
   h. Will my chosen health care provider still be able to deliver me?

    i. Will the baby have to stay in the hospital after delivery? If so, for how long?

    j. Can I meet with one or more specialists who have actually treated problems like the one(s) in my baby?

3. If the problem is chromosomal have your health care professional and/or the laboratory director meet with you to explain the results. Never allow a lab to give a result that is abnormal without interpretation. If a lab can not explain an abnormal chromosome report, you should seek a second opinion.

    a. Are all the cells abnormal or are there normal cells also? Ask to see an actual copy of the chromosomal karyotype report of your baby.

    b. Is this chromosomal abnormality lethal for the baby?

    c. Will the baby be retarded or brain impaired?

    d. Are there structural problems also associated with this abnormality?

    e. Ask how sure they are of the results? If they are not sure seek a second opinion.

    f. Are there any additional chromosomal studies or special tests that can be run to confirm the diagnosis? Would additional testing be helpful in making decisions?

4. Ask if there is a support group or society that you can talk with about other children that have had the same abnormalities?

5. Ask for the health care provider's personal experience of how these babies have done? Take this information as information only, since this is your baby not the health care provider's.

6. Never keep or end a pregnancy because a health care professional tells you to. You must make a decision that is right for you and your partner based upon the facts. We tell patients that it does not matter what we would do if we were in their situation because we are not in their situation. We can sympathize with you but we can not make a life and death decision for you. This is your pregnancy and you and/or your partner will have to live with the decision(s) that are made.

We call this field **Prenatal Diagnosis** which means that problems or abnormalities will hopefully be identified or detected, that problems will be evaluated and a prognosis and/or treatment plan developed. We feel that it is every expectant parent's duty to take an active role in finding out if there are any problems with their fetus and to take steps to give that child the best hope at a healthy future. As a consumer of medical services parents have a right to seek out and get enough information to make the right decision for them, since these decisions that are made during the pregnacy will stay with the parents and/or child for life.

TWINS/TRIPLETS ETC.

a. Are identical twins really identical?

Identical twins are the result of fertilization of one egg and one sperm with subsequent dividing and separation of the cells into two embryos. Once this division occurs each embryo forms separately. Therefore, even though both babies arise from a single egg and a single sperm, once the cells separate from each other, each embryos' cellular divisions that take place are not identical. It is believed that the earlier the separation takes place, the less similar the twins will be. Since both twins are a result of one egg and one sperm they will be more similar than fraternal twins.

Fraternal twins result from the fertilization of two different eggs with two different sperm. Identical twins occur by chance. Families can have an increased chance for fraternal twins. This occurs in some women who ovulate more than one egg per cycle even in the absence of fertility drugs. There are always extra sperm available to fertilize these "extra" eggs.

b. How can we determine if identical twins are identical?

If the sex of the babies are different they are not identical twins. If they look very different from each other they probably are not identical. To establish with certainty whether twins are identical or not, blood testing for red blood cell type, identifying "proteins" in the blood and determining the specific type of white blood cells the twins have, will confirm whether they are fraternal or identical.

ULTRASOUND

a. How long has ultrasound been used prenatally?

Ultrasound was first used for OB/GYN applications between 1965 and 1968 by a few research and university programs. Due to the poor image quality ultrasound was not believed to be an accurate diagnostic tool for prenatal diagnosis until the mid 1970's.

b. What is the risk of ultrasound in pregnancy?

To date, there have not be any published studies that have linked the use of ultrasound during pregnancy to any definite harm to the fetus. Ultrasound uses sound waves (not x-rays) to image the fetus. Initial studies which suggested the possible association between ultrasound and hearing or learning problems remain unsubstantiated. The ultrasound pictures that you see on the screen is a computer's interpretation of the sound waves that are bounced off the fetus.

c. How long has ultrasound been used with CVS or amniocentesis?

There are still well respected CVS and amniocentesis programs across the country that perform the procedures without the benefit of ultrasound guidance. However, most physicians that perform these procedures do use ultrasound to find a site to perform the procedure, guide the needle to the chorionic villi or amniotic fluid, and prevent the needle from coming in contact with the baby during the procedure. A miscarriage risk of 1:200-1:500 (0.20%-0.50%) following amniocentesis and approximately 1% for CVS was quoted for women who had the procedure without ultrasound guidance. There is not a national recommendation that CVS or amniocentesis be performed with ultrasound guidance. It is the physician's decision.

d. What is a Level II ultrasound?

A Level II ultrasound is a 30-45 minute targeted ultrasound to study the fetus and the pregnancy. This ultrasound is best performed between 15 and 18 weeks gestation. A Level II ultrasound includes a survey of the fetal anatomy either performed by a physician or read by a physician including:

1. Fetal head and its contents.
2. Fetal spine.
3. Kidneys.
4. Bladder.
5. Stomach.
6. Diaphragm.
7. Aortic arch.
8. 4 chamber view of the heart.
9. Right/left tibia and fibula.
10. Right/left femurs.
11. Right/left radius and ulna.
12. Number and position of fetus.
13. Placenta (location and integrity).
14. Umbilical cord insertion.
15. Number of vessels in the cord.
16. Volume of the amniotic fluid.
17. Posterior fossa (where the brain and spine come together).
18. Internal cervical os (opening of the uterus).
19. A general survery of the fetus for any irregularities, including hands and feet.

e. What can be determined by ultrasound during pregnancy?

1. Ultrasound can help an infertility patient determine how many follicles (eggs) she has during a cycle, and when she ovulates by monitoring the ovaries during the month.
2. Ultrasound performed between seven and nine weeks can help confirm the existence of an intrauterine preg-

nancy, the gestational weeks of the pregnancy, the number of fetuses and the viability of the fetus or fetuses.

3. It can help detect a tubal or ectopic pregnancy before it ruptures and injures the mother.

4. It can help evaluate the development of the fetus between 15 and 18 weeks gestation to help rule out physical abnormalities.

5. It can be used to help direct the needle for CVS, early amniocentesis or amniocentesis procedures.

6. The amniotic fluid volume can be monitored during the pregnancy to see if the fluid volume is too high (polyhydramnios), too low (oligohydramnios) or normal.

7. Ultrasound can be used to monitor the growth of fetuses that are either small or large for gestational age.

8. Physical abnormalities that are diagnosed between 15 and 18 weeks gestation can be monitored during the pregnancy to see if the abnormalities change or stay the same.

9. After 22 weeks gestation, the ultrasound can be used to reveal the chambers and vessels of the fetal heart. This is called fetal echocardiogram.

10. Ultrasound can monitor the well-being of the baby if the mother feels that the fetal movement is decreasing or she does not think the pregnancy feels "right".

11. Ultrasound can monitor the location of the placenta in relationship to the fetus so that a decision can be made ahead of time whether to try a normal vaginal delivery or schedule a C-section because of a placenta which lies low in the uterus or in front of the baby.

f. What is the difference between a two and three vessel cord?

As many as 20% of infants in pregnancy who have one umbilical artery rather than the normal two (a normal umbilical cord has two arteries and one vein) have congenital abnormalities making the risk approximately seven times higher than in fetuses with a normal three vessel cord. Male fetuses are more likely to have coincidental anomalies. The most common abnormalities found with a single umbilical artery include: cardiovascular malformations, neural tube and brain developmental abnormalities, genitourinary or gastrointestinal abnormalities and abdominal wall defect. There is also a higher risk of chromosomal abnormalities, particularly trisomies. In addition to the abnormalities described, perinatal mortality for these infants may approach 20% placing the pregnancy at high risk. Even when external anomalies are not identified, internal malformations may be present. Intrauterine growth retardation, which is common in these cases is usually corrected in the newborn period resulting in a near normal prognosis for infants whose only abnormal finding is a single umbilical artery.

Recommendations: A Level II ultrasound between 15 and 18 weeks gestation and a fetal echocardiogram after 22 weeks gestation is recommended for these fetuses and prenatal diagnosis by genetic amniocentesis is often suggested and performed.

g. What is a choroid plexus cyst?

With a remarkable improvement in technology for studying the fetus during pregnancy, choroid plexus cysts of the lateral ventricle of the brain may be detected in as many as 1:120 pregnancies when ultrasound imaging is performed between 15 and 20 weeks gestation. The choroid plexus cyst in the brain consists of blood vessels and supporting tissue and plays a role in the formation of cerebrospinal fluid.

The majority of these cysts resolve during the pregnancy or within several months after the delivery and present no risk to the baby. Occassionally, these cysts are found in infants with chromosomal abnormalities; primarily trisomy 18 and to a lesser degree trisomy 21 (Down syndrome). Rarely, other abnormalities including hydrocephalus (fluid on the brain), defects of the muscles of the abdominal wall, bladder or kidney abnormalities, cleft palate and heart defects are found in association with choroid plexus cysts. Choroid plexus cysts which are sausage shaped or larger than 10 mm, and those which are bilateral and the presence of other anatomical abnormalities are more likely to be significant to the fetus.

h. Why do I have to drink fluid before an ultrasound?

The reason why programs request that 12 ounces to 36 ounces of fluid (water, juice, tea etc.) be consumed 45 minutes to an hour before the ultrasound is performed is because a full bladder makes it easier to visualize the fetus and the uterus during the ultrasound study. If the bladder is not full enough to perform the study, you might have to be rescheduled. This fluid applies to transabdominal ultrasound studies only. A transvaginal ultrasound which uses a vaginal probe is preferred by many pregnant women because you do not need to have a full bladder to perform the study. Transvaginal ultrasound is primary used early in pregnancy when the fetus is too small to be seen abdominally or to look at the ovaries or cervix. The drawback of the transvaginal ultrasound is that as the baby develops it is usually too far away from the vaginal probe to be able to do an ultrasound study. Most programs try to use both transabdominal and transvaginal ultrasound studies depending upon the size of the baby, the weeks gestation of the pregnancy and how high or low the baby is in the uterus.

UMBILICAL CORD SAMPLING

a. What is umbilical cord sampling, when can it be performed and who can perform it?

Shortened terminology for percutaneous umbilical cord sampling (PUBS) is a procedure in which a needle is placed through the skin of the mother, the uterus and amniotic sac and then into one of the vessels in the umbilical cord. The blood specimen that is removed contains cells of the fetus. This test is used to confirm an unusual or abnormal finding from chorionic villus or amniotic fluid and can be used to study other diseases which might affect the fetus. The percutaneous umbilical cord sample can also be used to help detect certain disorders which may not be diagnosable by CVS or amniocentesis (e.g. If a chromosomal karyotype comes back from amniocentesis as being mosaic, the umbilical cord sampling can be used to try to find out if some or all of the cells are coming from the fetus or the placenta or both). Since PUBS allows the baby's blood cells to be analyzed rather than fetal cells that are found in amniotic fluid, the study is more accurate. It is similar to doing blood chromosomes on the baby once it is born. Since the test is performed on fetal blood, some labs can have results in 48-72 hours.

The reason that most women do not routinely have percutaneous umbilical cord sampling is that the miscarriage risk (approximately 2%-5% per procedure) is somewhat increased over CVS (1%-2%) or amniocentesis 1:200-1:500 (0.20%-0.50%). The PUBS procedure can be performed anytime during the pregnancy but is usually only performed when the risk to the baby from the abnormality or suspected problem is higher than the 2%-5% miscarriage risk. Also, the umbilical cord must be accessible. It is not always possible to sample the cord. The procedure is performed by a physician who specializes in complicated (high risk) pregnancies using ultrasound guidance. Many doctors who perform CVS or amniocentesis do not also perform the PUBS procedure. Usually these cases are referred by the CVS/amniocentesis specialist to a specialist who performs PUBS.

GLOSSARY OF ESSENTIAL GENETIC TERMS

AChE (Acetylcholinesterase): A protein found in the amniotic fluid that can be tested to help confirm an open neural defect or an abdominal wall defect.

AFP (Alphafetoprotein): A protein found in mother's blood and amniotic fluid. This protein level can help identify possible open neural tube defects, abdominal wall defects or pregnancies at an increased risk for Down syndrome.

AFP3 - The Triple Screen: A maternal blood test composed of three components (AFP, beta HCG and estriol) to help identify open neural tube defects or pregnancies at an increased risk for Down syndrome.

Amniocentesis: A procedure using a needle to remove fluid from the amniotic sac surrounding the fetus.

Artificial Insemination: An Assisted Reproductive technique to place sperm closer to an egg which has ovulated. The number and motility of sperm is enhanced in order to increase a patient's chance to conceive.

Autosomal Dominant: A mode of inheritance of a disease or trait which may approach 50%. Only one parent needs to have one abnormal gene for the baby to be affected.

Autosomal Recessive: A mode of inheritance of a disease in which the risk is 25% per pregnancy. Each parent would have to be a carrier of an abnormal gene for the baby to be affected.

Autosome: A chromosome other than a sex chromosome (X or Y), 22 pairs in humans.

Blood Chromosomes: A genetic analysis performed on the white blood cells of a patient.

Carrier: Usually refers to an individual who has one normal and one abnormal copy of a gene. If both copies were abnormal, a disease would be present (e.g. cystic fibrosis). For sex chromosomal abnormalities, if an abnormal X is inherited by a male who has only one X, a disease will be present (e.g. Hemophilia, Duchenne Muscular Dystrophy). A female with one normal and one abnormal X is a carrier.

Chorionic Villus Sampling: A procedure to remove placental cells very early in pregnancy (6-10 weeks) to study the chromosomes or enzymes of the fetus.

Chromosome: One of 46, divided into 23 pairs (numbered 1-22 and two sex chromosomes) found in every normal cell in the human body.

Chromosome disorder: A disorder due to an abnormal number of chromosomes, missing or extra parts of chromosomes, or possible unequal exchange of chromosomal material between chromosomes.

Congenital: Present at birth.

Cytogenetics: The study of cells in genetics. Includes studies of chromosomes.

Deletion: The loss of some DNA material from one or more chromosomes.

DNA: Deoxyribonucleic acid. The molecule responsible for transmitting genetic information.

Dominant: The presence of one copy of a gene is adequate for the presence of the gene to be recognized.

Donor Egg: An egg used to try to conceive a pregnancy that is obtained from a woman other than the mother of the baby.

Donor Sperm: Sperm used to try to conceive a pregnancy that is obtained from a man other than the father of the baby.

Familial: A trait or disorder which is more common in relatives from generation to generation than in the general population.

F.I.S.H.: (Fluorescent In Situ Hybridization): a technique to rapidly and accurately identify parts of or entire chromosomes from cells which are or are not dividing and which are living or preserved.

Gene: A specific sequence of DNA which results in a specific functional product.

Genetic Code: The genetic message which specifies the sequence of amnio acids necessary to synthesize a specific protein.

Genetic counseling: The process of acquisition of genetic family information to provide information regarding risks to individuals or familes for developing, transmitting, or preventing one or more disorders.

Genetic screening: Testing to identify individuals at risk for a specific disorder.

Genome: Complete DNA sequence of an individual species.

Genotype: Genetic constitution.

Gestation: Medical term for pregnant.

GIFT: Gamete (eggs and sperm) Intrafallopian Tube Transfer. An

Assisted Reproductive technique to help increase one's chances of conception by transfering eggs, mixed with sperm at the time of ovulation, surgically (laparoscopically) back into the fallopian tube.

Heritability: A statistical likelihood that a trait is genetically determined.

Human Genome Project: An international project to map the entire human genome (estimated 100,000 genes).

In-Utero: Inside the uterus, usually during pregnancy.

InVitro: An Assisted Reproductive technique to help fertilization: increases one's chances of conception by allowing sperm to fertilize one or more eggs outside the body (in a laboratory).

Karyotype: A pictorial representation of a person's chromosomes that allows them to be studied.

Meiosis: Cell division of the cells ultimately resulting in the production of an egg cell or sperm cell with 1/2 the chromosome number.

Mitosis: Cell division resulting in two cells genetically identical to the parent cell.

Mosaic: Two or more cell lines each with its own chromosomal composition.

Multifactorial: A mode of inheritance in which both genetic and environmental factors are involved.

Multiples of the Median: Refers to the range of values that may be seen in pregnancies with normal healthy babies. Values outside this range have a higher risk for abnormalities.

Mutation: A permanent change in a DNA sequence.

Neonatal: Newborn period.

Paternity Testing: Testing to attempt to determine the biological father of a child.

Pedigree: A pictorial representation of family members and their medical conditions; a family tree.

Preimplantation Genetics: Studies performed on a fertilized egg prior to its implantation in the uterus.

Prenatal: Before birth.

Prenatal Diagnosis: The attempt to identify possible physical and/or chromosomal abnormalities before birth.

Recessive: A disorder only expressed if it is present in two copies (one from each parent) or if it is the only active gene present (e.g. on an X chromosome in a male (XY)).

RNA: Ribonucleic acid; several types. Transfers message from nucleus DNA to direct protein synthesis.

Sex chromosomes: X or Y chromosomes. Females have two X chromosomes, males have one X and one Y.

Sex influenced: A trait expressed differently in males and females.

Sex limited: A trait expressed in one sex only.

Sex linked: (X-linked), old term used to describe traits on the X chromosome.

Translocation: When parts of one chromosome break off and exchange with another chromosome.

Ultrasound: The use of high frequency sound waves to create a picture of organs or tissues.

X-Linked: A mode of inheritance in which the abnormal gene is on one X chromosome.

X-Linked Disease: A disease which manifests itself in 50% of males who inherit the abnormal X. Females with one normal and one abnormal X are carriers.

ZIFT: Zygote Intrafallopian Tube Transfer. An Assisted Reproductive technique to help increase one's chances at conception by placing a fertilized egg (embryo) back into the fallopian tube.

PROFESSIONAL PROFILE
PAUL WEXLER, M.D.

We would like to thank Dr. Paul Wexler for editing this book. Dr. Wexler has done extensive work in the expanded applications of ultrasound studies in the pregnant patient and the use of diagnostic procedures such as CVS, early amniocentesis and amniocentesis. Working in conjunction with the University of Colorado Health Sciences Center on pregnant women in the late 1960's, Dr. Wexler took over the amniocentesis portion of the prenatal diagnosis program at the University of Colorado Health Sciences Center (UCHSC) in 1974 and remained in that capacity until 1980. In 1980, Dr. Wexler opened the Rose Medical Center Prenatal Diagnosis Program.

Dr. Wexler has performed in excess of 10,000 abdominal diagnostic procedures (including CVS, early amniocentesis and amniocentesis) during pregnancy. He has published more than 30 papers in the field of OB/GYN, including author of 5 chapters and co-editor of a well reviewed textbook entitled **Medical Care of the Pregnant Patient.**

Dr. Wexler did a postgraduate fellowship in Prenatal Genetics from 1981 until 1983. From 1990 until 1993, he served a second fellowship in clinical genetics at the University of Colorado Health Sciences Center/The Childrens' Hospital. He is currently on staff at the University of Colorado's Department of OB/GYN and the Division of Genetics at the Childrens' Hospital.

Dr. Wexler has been a physician in the Denver area since 1965. He received his B.A. degree in chemistry from the City College of New York in 1960. He went to medical school at the State University of New York - Downstate Medical Center in Brooklyn, New York from 1960 until 1964. After one year as a surgery intern at Kings County Hospital in Brooklyn, New York, he came to Colorado to train in OB/GYN at the University of Colorado. He served as a resident in OB/GYN from 1965 until 1967 and was chief resident from 1967 until 1968 in the Department of OB/GYN at the University of Colorado. He was board certified in OB/GYN in 1970.

While continuing to teach at the University of Colorado, he was in private practice from 1968 until 1974. In 1974, he left private practice to become an Assistant Clinical Professor in the Department of OB/GYN at the University of Colorado Health Sciences Center and Chairman of the Department of OB/GYN at Rose Medical Center. He remained Chairman of the Department of OB/GYN at Rose Medical Center until 1985 and advanced to the level of Clinical Professor of OB/GYN at the University of Colorado Health Sciences Center. He became Medical Director of Genassist Incorporated in 1983. He was President of the Colorado OB/GYN Society from 1984-1985.

A WORD ABOUT THE AUTHORS

KEITH WEXLER

Keith was born and raised in Denver, Colorado. He attended Littleton High School between 1980-1984. From 1984-1988 he attended Lewis and Clark College in Portland, Oregon where he received his Bachelor of Arts in International Affairs. In 1988, after graduation, Keith joined the Prenatal Diagnostic/Genetics Company, Genassist Incorporated located in Aurora, Colorado. In 1991, he was promoted to Vice President. He is still in that capacity today. He resides with his wife, Laurie and daughter, Haylee in Littleton, Colorado.

LAURIE NICHOLSON WEXLER

Laurie was born in Riverton, Wyoming. She attended Kelly Walsh High School in Casper, Wyoming between 1976-1980. From 1980-1982 she attended Casper College in Casper, Wyoming. From 1982-1984 she attended the University of Wyoming in Laramie, Wyoming where she received her Bachelor of Science in Zoology. Between 1984-1988 she attended Pacific University College of Optometry in Forest Grove, Oregon where she received her Optometry Doctorate. In 1988, she began private practice in Portland, Oregon as a Doctor of Optometry. From 1988-1989 she did an Optometry Teaching Fellowship. In 1991, she relocated her practice to Denver, Colorado. She is still in that capacity today. She resides with her husband, Keith and daughter, Haylee in Littleton, Colorado.

INDEX

FAMILY GENETIC PROFILE

We have included this form for you to use to obtain and organize your and/or your partner's medical history. Although a medical history form cannot detect all possible disorders that may affect you or your family members, the information you provide will help develop a more detailed picture of factors affecting your family. The **possibility** that you or other members of your family may develop certain medical conditions may be predicted with your help. The results of this history may indicate the need for further evaluation.

This form has been designed with great care so that it will be easy for you to understand and complete. Before completing the form, you may find it necessary to consult other members of your family to clarify details of your family's medical history.

This form is perforated so that you can make it available to your health care professional. If you have any questions about this form or how to fill it out, please call our office at 1-800-359-9412 between the hours of 8am and 5 pm (MST) Monday through Friday. **As with all medical history, this information will remain confidential.**

Patient Name: _____

Date of Birth: _____ Chronological Age: _____

Address: _____

_____

Telephone Number: _____ (Home) _____ (Work)

Partner's Name: _____

Date of Birth: _____ Chronological Age: _____

Doctor's Name and Address: _____

_____

Doctor's Telephone Number: _____

Insurance Company's Name and Address _____

_____

Insurance Company's Telephone Number _____

INSTRUCTIONS: Please complete this form by placing an "X" on each line that applies.

1. **Your Sex:**

    FEMALE: _____

    How many children have you had? _____

    Have you had previous genetic testing? Yes _____ No _____

    If yes, explain _____
    _____
    _____

    Have you had previous genetic couseling? Yes _____ No _____

    If yes, explain _____
    _____
    _____

    Are you pregnant now? Yes _____ No _____ If you are pregnant now:

    What was the first day of your last menstrual period? _____

    When is your due date? _____

    How many times have you been pregnant prior to now? _____
    (include miscarriages and abortions)

    How many children/live births have you had? _____

    How many documented spontaneous miscarriages have you had? _____

Have you ever had an "elective termination of pregnancy" (abortion)?

Yes _____ No _____

If yes, how many? _____

MALE: _____

How many children have you fathered? _____

Have you had previous genetic testing? Yes _____ No _____

If yes, explain _____

_____

_____

_____

Have you had previous genetic counseling? Yes _____ No _____

If yes, explain _____

_____

_____

_____

2. **Are you and your spouse/partner related (i.e. do you have blood relatives in common)?**

If yes, specify who: _____

_____

_____

_____

_____

_____

3. **Are you or spouse/partner adopted?** Yes _____ No _____

If yes, specify who: _____

_____

_____

_____

_____

4. **What is your ethnic/racial background? (Some inherited diseases are more common in certain ethnic/racial groups.)**

	SELF	PARTNER
Black	_____	_____
Caucasian	_____	_____
Jewish (ethnicity)	_____	_____
Mediterranean (Greek, Italian)	_____	_____
Oriental/Asian	_____	_____
Hispanic/Chicano/Central or South American	_____	_____

Other, or combinations of above: (Specify) _____

_____

_____

_____

Does anyone in your family, or do you or your partner have any of the following?
*Include any previous partners with whom you have had children.
*DO NOT include those who have been adopted.

1. **Infertility (Difficulty becoming pregnant for more than 6 months.)**

   Yes _____ No _____ Who _____

   Describe _____

   _____

   _____

   _____

   _____

2. **More than one miscarriage and/or loss of baby.**

   Yes _____ No _____ Who _____

   Describe _____

   _____

   _____

3. History of diabetes and/or diabetes during pregnancy.

Yes _____ No _____ Who _____

Describe _____
_____
_____
_____
_____

4. History of rapid or "painless" labor and/or premature birth.

Yes _____ No _____ Who _____

Describe _____
_____
_____
_____
_____

5. History of a stillborn infant and/or child that died shortly after birth. (Include SIDS/Sudden Infant Death Syndrome).

Yes _____ No _____ Who _____

Describe _____
_____
_____
_____
_____

6. History of medical difficulties during the newborn period.

Yes _____ No _____ Who _____

Describe _____
_____
_____
_____

7. **Developmental Delay (i.e. motor, speech, etc.) or Learning Problems.**

   Yes _____ No _____ Who _____

   Describe _____
   _____
   _____
   _____
   _____

8. **Mental Retardation.**

   Yes _____ No _____ Who _____

   Describe _____
   _____
   _____
   _____
   _____

9. **Chronic Psychiatric, Psychological, Emotional and Behavioral Problems.**

   Yes _____ No _____ Who _____

   Describe _____
   _____
   _____
   _____
   _____

10. **Brain Abnormality/Anencephaly/Fluid on the Brain (Hydrocephalus).**

    Yes _____ No _____ Who _____

    Describe _____
    _____
    _____
    _____
    _____

11. **Deafness/Ear Abnormalities.**

Yes _____ No _____ Who _____

Describe _____
_____
_____
_____
_____

12. **Blindness/Eye Abnormalities.**

Yes _____ No _____ Who _____

Describe _____
_____
_____
_____
_____

13. **Lip/Mouth Deformity.**

Yes _____ No _____ Who _____

Describe _____
_____
_____
_____
_____

14. **Cleft Palate/Cleft Lip.**

Yes _____ No _____ Who _____

Describe _____
_____
_____
_____

15. **Skin Abnormalities.**

Yes _____ No _____ Who _____

Describe _____
_____
_____
_____
_____

16. **Spine Deformity/Spina Bifida.**

Yes _____ No _____ Who _____

Describe _____
_____
_____
_____
_____

17. **Bone Deformity.**

Yes _____ No _____ Who _____

Describe _____
_____
_____
_____
_____

18. **Hand/Feet Abnormalities.**

Yes _____ No _____ Who _____

Describe _____
_____
_____
_____
_____

19. **Club Foot.**

    Yes _____ No _____ Who _____

    Describe _____
    _____
    _____
    _____
    _____

20. **Heart Defect/Hole in Heart.**

    Yes _____ No _____ Who _____

    Describe _____
    _____
    _____
    _____
    _____

21. **Heart Attack Before Age 50.**

    Yes _____ No _____ Who _____

    Describe _____
    _____
    _____
    _____
    _____

22. **Seizures/Epilepsy/Convulsions/"Fits".**

    Yes _____ No _____ Who _____

    Describe _____
    _____
    _____
    _____
    _____

23. **Muscle/Nerve Disorder.**

Yes _____ No _____ Who _____

Describe _____

_____

_____

_____

_____

24. **Polycystic Kidneys/Horseshoe Kidneys.**

Yes _____ No _____ Who _____

Describe _____

_____

_____

_____

_____

25. **Bleeding Disorders.**

Yes _____ No _____ Who _____

Describe _____

_____

_____

_____

_____

26. **Cystic Fibrosis.**

Yes _____ No _____ Who _____

Describe _____

_____

_____

_____

_____

27. **Asthma/Severe Allergies.**

 Yes _____ No _____ Who _____

 Describe _____
 _____
 _____
 _____
 _____

28. **PKU/Phenylketonuria.**

 Yes _____ No _____ Who _____

 Describe _____
 _____
 _____
 _____
 _____

29. **Hypothyroidism/Hyperthyroidism (Low/High Thyroid Function).**

 Yes _____ No _____ Who _____

 Describe _____
 _____
 _____
 _____
 _____

30. **Thalassemia/Blood Disorder.**

 Yes _____ No _____ Who _____

 Describe _____
 _____
 _____
 _____
 _____

31. **Hemophilia.**

Yes _____ No _____ Who _____

Describe _____

_____

_____

_____

_____

32. **Sickle Cell Disease or Trait.**

Yes _____ No _____ Who _____

Describe _____

_____

_____

_____

_____

Have you been tested for Sickle Cell Disease?

Yes _____ No _____ Results _____

Has your partner been tested for Sickle Cell Disease?

Yes _____ No _____ Results _____

33. **Tay Sachs Disease.**

Yes _____ No _____ Who _____

Describe _____

_____

_____

_____

_____

Have you been tested for Tay Sachs Disease?

Yes _____ No _____ Results _____

Has your partner been tested for Tay Sachs Disease?

Yes _____ No _____ Results _____

34. **Are you or your partner taking any prescription medication for any medical disease (e.g. high blood pressure etc? Specify name of drug if known).**

Yes _____ No _____ Who _____

Describe _____
_____
_____
_____
_____

35. **Diagnosed genetic (inherited) diseases not mentioned?**

Yes _____ No _____ Who _____

Describe _____
_____
_____
_____
_____

36. **Are there any other serious specific disorders, conditions, or unusual traits that run in your family or your partner's family about which you are concerned?**

Yes _____ No _____

If yes, describe _____
_____
_____
_____

37. **Have you had a fever during this pregnancy?**

If yes, please explain _____
_____
_____
_____

38. **Have you had any vaccinations during this pregnancy?**

   If yes, please explain _____

   _____

   _____

   _____

39. **Is this pregnancy the result of insemination with donor sperm or egg?**

   If yes, explain _____

   _____

   _____

   _____

40. **Is this pregnancy a result of Assisted Reproductive Techniques (e.g. drugs, manipulation of eggs or sperm; GIFT, ZIFT or In-Vitro)?**

   If yes, explain _____

   _____

   _____

   _____

   Have you or your partner been exposed to any of the following: (CHECK IF USED DURING THIS PREGNANCY)

41. **Prescription Drugs**

   You _____ Your Partner _____
   Describe _____

   _____

   _____

   _____

42. **Over-the-Counter Drugs (i.e. aspirin, laxatives, sleeping pills, cold tablets, weight control medicine etc.)**

   You _____ Your Partner _____
   Describe _____

   _____

   _____

   _____

43. Recreational Drugs (i.e. Marijuana, Cocaine, LSD, etc.)

   You _____ Your Partner _____
   Describe _____
   _____
   _____

44. Environmental Agents (i.e. chemicals, cleaning agents, etc. at home or work).

   You _____ Your Partner _____
   Describe _____
   _____
   _____

45. Alcohol:

   Less than one mixed drink, one glass of wine, or one beer/day?

   You _____ Partner _____ Describe _____

   One mixed drink, two glasses of wine or two beers/day?

   You _____ Partner _____ Describe _____

   Three mixed drinks, or three glasses of wine or three beers/day?

   You _____ Partner _____ Describe _____

   More than three mixed drinks, or three glasses of wine or three beers/day?

   You _____ Partner _____ Describe _____

CHECK IF USED DURING THIS PREGNANCY:

46. Cigarettes:

   Less than one-half pack per day?

   You _____ Partner _____ Describe _____

One to two packs per day?

You _____ Partner _____ Describe _____

More than two packs per day?

You _____ Partner _____ Describe _____

47. **X-rays:**

You _____ Partner _____

Describe _____

_____

_____

48. **Are you or your partner being followed by a specialty physician for any chronic disease or condition?**

You _____ Partner _____

Describe _____

_____

_____

The ABC's of Prenatal Diagnosis

ORDER FORM

Single or multiple copies of this book may be ordered by sending $7.00 per copy, check or money order payable to:

Genassist Incorporated
c/o ABC
2530 S. Parker Road #405
Aurora, CO 80014

Please mail the copy or copies to the following address or addresses:

_____

_____

_____

_____

We encourage you to tell us what you think of this book? Comments and/or criticisms are welcomed. Are there chapters or questions that were not in the book that you would like included? Please complete below or attach additional pages if necessary. We will respond.

_____

_____

_____

_____

_____

_____

_____